The Catholic Physician:
Messages from the Spiritual Advisor

Other books by the authors:

Seven Minute Homilies, 2017
Msgr. Dino Lorenzetti
Available from: St. John the Baptist School, 716.877.6401

Addio: See You in Heaven, 2016*
Msgr. Dino Lorenzetti & Barbara Stoyell-Mulholland

The Agony of Betrayal, 2015*
Msgr. Dino Lorenzetti & Barbara Stoyell-Mulholland

Mavourneen, 2013*
Barbara Stoyell-Mulholland

Books are available on Lulu.com

The Catholic Physician: Messages from the Spiritual Advisor

Msgr. Dino Lorenzetti

Edited by: Barbara Stoyell-Mulholland

2021

The authors wish to allow printing and copying of this book for the purpose of sharing God's good news to his people.

This book can be ordered from Lulu.com

100% of the proceeds from this book will be donated to the Catholic Medical Association in honor of all physicians who listen to the call of Christ.

Copyright © 2021 by Barbara Stoyell-Mulholland

ISBN 978-1-105-57616-4

First Printing: 2021

Dedication

To the physicians who so inspired me

physician[1]
noun

phy·si·cian | \ fə-ˈzi-shən \
Definition of *physician*

1: a person skilled in the art of healing *specifically*: one educated, clinically experienced, and licensed to practice medicine as usually distinguished from surgery

2: one exerting a remedial or salutary influence

---

[1] From Merriam-Webster dictionary

Table of Contents

A Message from the Editor..1

The Latest Message from Msgr. Lorenzetti................3

Section 1: Who is the Catholic Physician?..................5

    The Unseen Qualities of a Catholic Physician..........7

    Listening to the Divine Healer...................................9

    Living the Gospel Message.......................................11

    As an Imitator of Christ..13

    Becoming a Eucharistic Physician...........................15

    Working with the Divine Physician.........................19

    The Physician's Hands..21

    The Physician's Eyes: "Faith Vision".......................23

    Dedicating Yourself to the Kingdom.......................25

    The Physician and the Mystical Body of Christ......27

    As a Priestly Vocation...29

    Beneficiaries of His Largesse...................................31

    The Clown of Godspell..35

    Yes, Lord, I Will Serve..37

    The Mystery of a Vocation.......................................39

Section 2: Be Inspired by Scripture..........................41

    We Are Tenants in the Vineyard.............................43

There Are No Small Gestures: Veronica, Simon, & Dismas.. 47

Physicians as Innkeepers.. 49

On Being a Prudent and Vigilant Bridesmaid Awaiting the King 51

Physician as Shepherd: Psalm 23 53

Observing Mary.. 55

Sirach Extols the Physician 57

Section 3: Practicing the Practice 59

Fasting and Praying Before Practice 61

Seeking Solutions Through Petition......................... 63

Protecting Yourself From Anxiety 65

Fatigue 67

Happiness Is… 69

Physician, You Are Healed 71

Searching for the Holy: For You................................ 73

Discouragement with Patients 75

The Redemptive Physician/Patient Relationship .. 77

We Are Created in the Image of God........................ 79

Section 4: Suffering and Healing 81

Jesus Experienced Death.. 83

Violence and the Author of Life................................. 85

[x]

The Destructive Power of Rejection 87
Curing With Words 89
Suffering and Success 91
The Supernatural Power of Healing 93
Our Disease: Lack of Self-Worth 95

Section 5: What is Truth in a Secular Society? 97
Courage in a Secular Society 99
Truth and the Physician 101
Apostolic Mission on the Right to Life 103
The Value of Life 105
The Absolute Evil of Abortion 107
Hero or Scapegoat? 109
Pragmatism May Facilitate Evil 111
Obstacles in Legal Regulations 113
Working Toward a Dream: Medicine and the Law
.... 115

About the Author 119

A Message from the Editor

I am confident I met Msgr. Dino Lorenzetti when I was an infant and during my toddler years. My parents were heavily involved in Foundation for International Cooperation (FIC) and Family Life in the Diocese of Buffalo, NY. But I have no recollections of these get-togethers.

However, as I was growing up, my mom (my dad passed years ago) spoke often and fondly of Fr. Dino. I, and all of my ten siblings, moved out of the Buffalo area and my mom retired to Florida. In the few years before my mom died, she asked if I would take her to visit the "retired" Fr. Dino when we traveled to Buffalo. It was during these visits I was introduced to the vibrant, funny, compassionate, and reverent Fr. Dino.

When he discovered and read a memoir I had written for my mother, he became intrigued with the idea of sharing and writing about a recent experience that had transformed him. Fr. Dino enlisted my help and *The Agony of Betrayal* was born. Since then, I have joyfully worked on a number of writing projects with him. His keen insight, humility, acute sense of humor, and wisdom from almost 100 years of living has captivated me, as it does with almost everyone he encounters.

A couple of years ago, Fr. Dino asked me if his 20+ years of reflections for Catholic physicians were worthwhile preserving and sharing with today's physicians. After reviewing his writings on the subject, I was reminded why Truth is eternal. His words, written in the 60's, 70's, and 80's, are as true today as on the days they were first written. My editing primarily consisted of updating language and bringing out related themes.

May Fr. Dino's words bless you and your vocation as they have blessed the physicians who read them in years past.

Barbara Stoyell-Mulholland
Baltimore, MD

"The sick are privileged for the Church, for the priestly heart, for all the faithful. They are not to be discarded. On the contrary, they are to be healed, to be cared for. They are the object of Christian concern."

~ Pope Francis
General Audience
August 28, 2019

The Latest Message from Msgr. Lorenzetti

From the earliest of ages, men and women who healed the sick were looked upon with great dignity and respect. Physicians, even to this day, are seen as persons of dignity and nobility and their vocation is listed among the greatest bestowed on us. This vocation mirrors Jesus' ministry of healing the sick, comforting the dying and, as Divine Physician, assuring all who have faith in Him "even when they die, live."

There exists an intimate relationship of the physician with the divine: the doctor, realizing his/her limitations, relies on the Creator for guidance, wisdom, and the gift of healing.

For decades I was the Spiritual Advisor for the Catholic Medical Association (previously known as the National Federation of Catholic Physicians' Guilds) and as the Ecclesiastical Assistant to the International Federation of Catholic Medical Associations under Pope St. Paul VI and Pope St. John Paul II. While working alongside the medical community during this time, this is what I learned:

- *SCIENCE:* I was taught the science behind Natural Family Planning which helped with my work in the Family Life Department.
- *INSPIRATION:* The undeterred dedication of those in the medical profession was inspiring to me: watching their willingness to care for

the sick, reach out to the poor, and to teach our young adults preparing for marriage.
- *FAITH:* It was humbling to witness their prayer life, their trust in the Divine Physician for assistance, and their Mass attendance and hope in the Eucharist.
- *FAMILY:* I was taught serving the sick includes concern for the patient's family
- *GENEROSITY OF THE GOOD SAMARITAN:* I was reminded each patient was made in the image and likeness of God. Physicians gave patients their best, even if the patient didn't have the financial means, or even if it was not their preference.
- *AVAILABLITY:* Physicians taught me that our service to the Lord is night or day and is never constrained by so-called office hours.

As Spiritual Advisor of the CMA from 1967 to 1988, I was invited by the *Linacre Quarterly* to write messages for the Catholic physician. Truth stands the test of time and now years later, as I near my 100th birthday, and encouraged by others, I offer updated reflections from these, and other publications, to you. I also wish to express my gratitude to Barbara Stoyell-Mulholland for making this book a reality. Her professionalism and additions to my writings will be forever appreciated. With God's grace, may these readings help to enrich your vocation of healing and ministering to the sick and the dying.

Mgr. Dino Lorenzetti, July 2021

Section 1: Who is the Catholic Physician?

The Unseen Qualities of a Catholic Physician[1]

When meeting a Catholic physician, there is much more to that person than meets the eye. This is like observing a crescent moon and being aware that there is more to that satellite than what radiates to earth. The unseen qualities of the physician of faith include a lifestyle of prayer, a willingness to heal for the glory of God, and to be an instrument of grace proclaiming the Gospel message as a prophet of Christ.

A doctor is the beloved of God and can tie in with His divinity. In doing so, the greater part remains unseen, yet ever present.

In the Liturgy of the Eucharist, the priest-celebrant prays at the Offertory as he blesses the water (representing you and me) into the cup filled with wine (representing Christ), saying these words: "By the mystery of the water and wine, may we come to share in the divinity of Christ, who humbled Himself to share in our humanity."

The oneness of the physician with Jesus becomes a consecrated unity. Through the Spirit of the Lord, miracles of healing take place in the patient's mind and body as your sacrament is administered in His name. Your services, smiles, and words give hope to the sick person and have a healing effect on you, the

---

[1] Lorenzetti, Dino (1988) "Message From the Spiritual Advisor," The Linacre Quarterly: Vol. 55: No. 1, Article 2

physician, as you are healed through these acts of mercy.

The power of God's grace enlightens and strengthens all that you do. Having been selected as an instrument of God's love, you too are called to expel unclean spirits, calm fevers, and restore the sick to the fullness of health. In union with the invisible God, the Holy Spirit shines through you and your (His) works, and thus the Father is glorified.

One may ask, "Who is a Catholic physician?" The response from a person of faith would declare him or her to be a dedicated doctor, competent, being in union with Christ and His Church, who prays, forgives, respects life, and is always willing to help those in need.

What an honor to hold such a sacred office! Yes, the Catholic physician has been especially chosen to be one in Christ. It is indeed a blessing to be so gifted in this vocation.

God has set you apart: "To me, therefore, you shall be holy; for I, the Lord, am holy, and I have set you apart from other peoples to be my own."[2]

---

[2] Lev 20:26

Listening to the Divine Healer[1]

The Catholic physician, by the very title, is someone more than a doctor: someone who is a specialist in curing the sick, a respected person in the community, and a learned individual. Through baptism, the physician is given a special commission, indelibly marked in the person which is inseparable from the profession. The Catholic physician is to bring the Light of Christ to patients.

Primitive cultures feared two great evils: sickness and darkness. Sickness was the unknown enemy that destroyed the body from within and darkness helped the enemy to destroy the body from without. With both, the community was endangered.

Yet, ancient cultures associated life with light. With the warmth of the sun, plants took life, and in the brightness of the day, the enemy was seen so life could be protected from the aggressor.

The medical doctor has always been recognized as a person of vision, gifted with knowledge, artistic ability, and natural talents. This profession also trains the medical student to discern the darkness of disease and with learned skills, assist the community to greater health and life.

During His public life, Christ, the Divine Physician and "light of the world," restored sight to the blind,

---

[1] Lorenzetti, Dino J. (1967) "The Catholic Physician," The Linacre Quarterly: Vol. 34: No. 3, Article 41.

health to the sick, and knowledge to the ignorant. In His love for us, He inspired those who wished to follow Him in the Way, the Truth, and the Life. Truth can be lived when the "enlightened" Catholic physician lives in a Christ-like manner, serving God the Father, through the inspiration of the Holy Spirit, to assist His people walking in the darkness of sickness and sin.

The Catholic physician, striving for perfection in this vocation, should listen to the voice of the Divine Healer. In so doing, the doctor becomes conscious, through the light of Christ, of the needs of the community crying not only from physical pain but also from economic, social, and psychological sufferings. The healer becomes sensitized to the needs of each individual who has a soul that will live for eternity. Each patient is a person with a specific need, rather than a chart or "case number." For some, the Catholic physician responds with words of comfort; others may need guidance through a critical stage; and still others need clarity when tangled with necessary medical and governmental forms.

Every client needs the doctor's time, patience, and love. When this is accomplished, then the words of Christ will re-echo, "Amen, I say to you, whatever you did for one of these least brothers of mine, you did for me."[2] May God reward the Catholic physician's response to His people, and grant life eternal for dedicated service.

---

[22] Mt 25:40

Living the Gospel Message[1]

We are not born EQUAL, except in dignity. Surely, no one can question we are all different: men and women; rich and poor; sick and healthy; varied talents. Yet, each is called to the new life God has prepared for us. We are called to love, helping one another to arrive at our true home: Paradise.

When Jesus spoke on the Mount, He taught His disciples how this can be done. The reward is great for those poor in spirit, the lowly, the merciful, the single-hearted, and the peacemakers. He extolled the child-like: humble, loving, and willing to serve. These are more assured of the Kingdom than the proud, boastful, powerful, and selfish.

Jesus defined love when he said, "No one has greater love than this, to lay down one's life for one's friends."[2] Relatively few are invited to heroically die for another. However, all of us are called to surrender our lives. Our lives, essentially, consist of time; there are just so many hours, days, and years until the august audience before the throne of God. Therefore, when we spend an hour with a patient – with anyone – we have shared an hour of our life, an hour of our love; we have died with that individual as we have lived in Christ.

---

[1] EXCERPTS from Msgr. Lorenzetti Homily at XIV World Congress of the International Federation of Catholic Medical Associations. Mumbai, India, January 29, 1978. St. Mother Theresa was present and signed a copy of this homily.
[2] Jn 15:13

The secular world can equate time with money; but those living the Gospel equate time with eternity. Those who love God give themselves to prayer, care for the needs of others, comfort the disturbed, heal the sick, and share gifts and talents so that others may enjoy a better life. This is pleasing to the Lord.

When Lazarus died, Jesus went to the tomb and raised him back to life. The apostle John tells us that it was from "that day then, they planned to kill Him."[3] In bringing the restored quality of life back to his friend, Jesus paid the price of love.

The prophet Zephaniah wrote that God "will leave a remnant in your midst, a people humble and lowly who shall take refuge in the name of the Lord."[4] YOU are that remnant who believe in Him and place your trust in His love. YOU are the sign of the contradiction to the secular world; your success, in spite of great obstacles, has been your faith, your confidence in the Lord, your professionalism, and your love for your patients. In uniting yourself to God's will, He has rewarded you with courage and strength.

When living your mission of living the Gospel, then, be not concerned if you are criticized, insulted, or persecuted, for Jesus assures you: "Rejoice and be glad, for your reward will be great in heaven."[5]

---

[3] Jn 11: 53
[4] Zep 3:12
[5] Mt 5:12

As an Imitator of Christ[1]

The vocation of the Catholic physician parallels the life of Christ in many ways, including His miracles of healing and His sufferings in restoring the sinner to new life.

St. John says that our Lord Jesus, on His journey from Judea to Galilee, rested at Jacob's well in Samaria and asked the woman with "five husbands" for a drink, assuring her that if she only knew what God gives, she would ask for and receive living water and eternal life.[2] The physician – likewise fatigued and exhausted – is like an "oasis" in the desert, refreshing the patient "dehydrated" in health, healing with loving care, offering hope and new life.

Perhaps the most exasperating period in the physician's life is the ongoing temptation of discouragement and the desire to "give up" or "get away from it all." Sometimes the urge to retire, avoid the madness of governmental bookkeeping, relieve the unnecessary harassment from society, or to escape excessive taxation and insurance premiums seems to be the most sensible solution to daily problems. Like Christ, we are tempted by Satan to admit defeat and to surrender. However, Jesus told Satan "to be gone" for His mission was to do the will of His Father, to

---

[1] Lorenzetti, Dino J. (1976) "The Catholic Physician ... An Imitator of Christ," The Linacre Quarterly: Vol. 43: No. 2, Article 2.
[2] Jn 4

redeem mankind, and to give new life to those dead in sin.

And so, be encouraged as you journey through counseling and compassion, through medication and X-rays, through anesthesia and surgery – all with the hope of redeeming the sick to new life.

In His passion and death, Jesus is apparently rewarded with rebuke, ridicule, and abandonment from the very ones to whom He gave life. How often can you identify with our Lord as you dedicate your services of love, with the best of your talents, and find yourself faced with a disgruntled patient or even a malpractice lawsuit?

Be inspired by Jesus: as a teacher, a model of holiness manifesting patience, compassion, kindness, and sensitivity to the needs of His people. For you, too, live a vocation (on and off duty) by inspiring others, giving witness of your faith to patients, students, nurses, interns, parents, and children alike. This is what it truly means to be Christ-like: a Christian hero in these most troublesome times.

What the world needs NOW are persons who believe, who are committed, willing to give totally and lovingly. As every Christian is, the Catholic physician is also called upon to be perfected in holiness.

Becoming a Eucharistic Physician[1]

To be a Catholic physician in today's society, one is usually an unsung hero, upholding high values of the vocation, and confronting the challenges of pragmatism, which encourage the disposal of anything unwanted.

To be this ideal physician, it becomes necessary not only to be *close* to Christ, but in fact *united* with Him. St. Luke, the physician and evangelist, tells us that when Jesus was in the synagogue on the sabbath to teach, He restored the withered right hand of a man. The Scribes and Pharisees were filled with fury, and began to discuss among themselves what they should do to Jesus. The very next sequence in the Scriptures shows Jesus "went out to the mountain to pray." [2]

The Catholic physician, imitating Jesus, must find time in the course of a hectic day to retreat from the vocation of healing and go to pray – be refreshed, renewed, strengthened – so as to continue the apostolate of imitating Christ.

A physician I knew was once asked by some local medical students: "When do you find time to pray?" His answer is worth reflecting for he said, "My whole life is a prayer." He continued by telling these students that when he examines his conscience, should he find that

---

[1] Lorenzetti, Dino J. (1978) "Message From the Spiritual Advisor," The Linacre Quarterly: Vol. 45: No. 2, Article 2
[2] Lk 6:11-12

he was selfish or working for the wrong objectives, he asks God for forgiveness and strength so that he may do better the following day.

Many years ago, I was fortunate to attend the XIV World Congress of the International Federation of Catholic Medical Associations with St. Mother Teresa of Kolkata. Mother Teresa told this story from her many daily experiences:

> A woman who was dying on one of the many busy streets in India was picked up to prepare for death. I asked myself, "I wonder what I would say if I were she? Would I have complained about the way I was treated – not having been given food, medicine, clothing, or shelter?" While reflecting on these personal thoughts, the woman looked at me lovingly, said "Thank you," and died. Her very last breath was a gift – she gave all she had.

"Thanks" is an abbreviation for the word Thanksgiving, which means Eucharist. The Catholic physician is a Eucharistic physician, literally consumed, giving totally in love for God's people. In the Eucharist, Jesus shares an intimacy with His loved ones and the Eucharistic physician does the same. This consumed life becomes a living symbol, a sacramental sign, not apart from the people, but stands out among them. Jesus said "This is My Body – given up for you." Is not the Eucharistic doctor doing likewise? By living this vocation, witness is given to the reality of Christian love.

Becoming a Eucharistic physician does not happen overnight. This growth does not occur by one's willing it. It must be worked out, being put to the test, being subject to ridicule or persecution; it is sacrificial and could involve loss: personal, social, or financial.

Faith is something more than simply listening to the Word of God; it is an investment of total surrender to Christ's love. Being conscious of this, the physician must continue with self-reflection and examination of actions. For if one is dwelling in love of Christ, this blessing can be assured:

> "If you remain in me and my words remain in you, ask for whatever you want and it will be done for you. By this is my Father glorified, that you bear much fruit and become my disciples. As the Father loves me, so I also love you. Remain in my love."[3]

The Eucharistic physician may not be looked upon as a "winner" in the eyes of the world. But those who have faith know differently.

---

[3] Jn 15:7-9

Working with the Divine Physician[1]

Healing is at the heart of a physician's ministry. At times, its mystery perplexes even the most sophisticated scholar, for its source is often unknown. Every experienced examiner can cite numerous cases where a patient has complained of pain, discomfort, or even severe illness and then, without the physician ever knowing why, the patient is cured or "healed." The question goes unanswered as to whether the ailment was caused by physical, spiritual, or emotional sickness, and while no one seems to be given credit for the phenomenon, still the reality exists.

In a pragmatic society, the Catholic physician recognizes God is the source of all life and that the physician facilitates His divine plan. United with Jesus Christ through Baptism and the Eucharist, the doctor has the power of Christ within, like the woman with the hemorrhage in the Gospel story[2] who only needed to touch Jesus' garment and His power flowed into her, thus restoring her to new life. God's grace can flow through your personal touch.

It is well known that patients often wait long, anxious hours to see and hear what the physician has to say about their health. They are eager to listen to every word uttered, for their future may be revealed in "what the doctor has to say." It is here that the personal touch

---

[1] Lorenzetti, Dino J. (1979) "Message From the Spiritual Advisor," The Linacre Quarterly: Vol. 46: No. 2, Article 2
[2] Lk 8:43-44

of the prayerful physician, with child-like faith and confidence, can uplift the sick person. As a mediator of the healing power of Jesus Christ, those in pain and illness can be helped through this special sacrament of love.

Speaking in faith over the sick, a positive action takes place. Through God's amazing grace, tense anxieties locked in the deep recesses of the troubled patient's very being are often freed, and the words of love by the physician bring healing and peace.

The label "Catholic" branded on a doctor in a secular society may seem to be a handicap, yet as the physician practices medical skills which are spiritually enriched with God's love, patients become doubly blessed. They are being treated by a person who not only has expertise in medicine, but who is also continuing the mission of healing as Jesus did – God working "with him, in him and through him" (or her, as the case may be).

Doctors, do not ever underestimate your power. You are special people, chosen by God to be His "messengers." For being one with Him, the impossible becomes possible.

The Physician's Hands[1]

While meditating on the life of Jesus, one could easily visualize His tender hands as a small child, His muscular hands as a carpenter, His physician hands when healing, and His pierced hands after being nailed to the cross.

St. John tells us that Thomas was not with the apostles when Jesus first appeared to them and he did not believe Jesus rose. Eight days later, with the doors closed, Jesus came, stood in their midst, and said to Thomas, "Put your finger here and see my hands, and bring your hand and put it into my side, and do not be unbelieving, but believe."[2]

The pierced hands of Jesus were shown to the Father after His resurrection from the grave and they remain as a memorial of His crucifixion.

Every hand tells a story, especially the one that was pierced. There are those who falsely claim to read the future from the palms of one's hands. A calloused hand has the experience of hard labor. An artist's hands bring to life the very beauty of the soul.

The physician, who touches life itself, uses her hands for restoring to the fullness of life the dormant body, weakened through sickness and disease.

---

[1] Lorenzetti, Dino (1980) "Message From the Spiritual Advisor," The Linacre Quarterly: Vol. 47: No. 1, Article
[2] Jn 20:27

In the course of a busy day, the physician puts two willing hands to many uses – examining the body, performing surgery, handling delicate instruments, writing prescriptions, stitching the patient, and comforting families. At a delivery, with strong hands, an obstetrician may handle the new life at birth, ensure the new intake of breath, congratulate the parents, and pray in thanksgiving. The physician always continues the mission of Jesus in healing the sick through science, art, and the *imposition of hands*.

A positive mark of Catholic physicians is that their hands are never used in an act of violence. The sacredness of the very person is upheld, including the physician's sacred life, and hands are always extended to praise God, preserve life, and help the neighbor in pain. In union with Jesus at the baptism in the Jordan, as well as at death at Calvary, special strength is found by knowing the physician's hands, too, are nailed to the cross of Christ. Our gifted hands are not free to be used for secular gain, but only to do the will of the Father.

Unlike St. Francis of Assisi or St. Padre Pio, the stigmata of the Catholic physician is invisible. The stigmata is painful: yet as many suffer the pain, they will also share in the ultimate of glory with Him in whom the Father is well pleased. The physician of faith finds that the mission field is Christ-centered, the work is holy, hands are sacred, and the reward is Resurrection.

The Physician's Eyes: "Faith Vision"[1]

Physicians are called to "see" problems and ailments, often invisible disorders which are causing pain, discomfort, and sickness. The human eye frequently can detect the abnormality, but more often than not, it is left up to the doctor to determine the unseen cause of the issues.

Catholic physicians must look even deeper into what ails their patients. This "faith vision" enables them to see the hidden strengths and weaknesses of their patients and to direct them toward new avenues of recovery.

While an eagle has extraordinary sharpness of vision so it can see a lizard resting on a rock some thousand feet below, the human eye is certainly not expected to view such distant objects with precision. People of faith have vision which enables them to see goodness in others, to understand strength in compassion, to radiate courage and, above all, to rely on the healing power of God's love.

Upon meeting Jesus, many saints, and the apostles in particular, felt compelled to "leave all and follow Him." Encountering His magnetism and His holiness gave them the inspiration to leave their former style of life, pick up their cross daily and, if necessary, accept death

---

[1] Lorenzetti, Dino J. (1983) "Message from the Spiritual Advisor: Physicians' 'Faith Vision'," The Linacre Quarterly: Vol. 50: No. 3, Article 2

for Him. They saw something in Christ to which others were blinded.

These so-called ordinary people with extraordinary vision were, perhaps, looked upon in their day as unimportant citizens, yet they turned out to be the heroes of the Church. They displayed the power of the divine Spirit which transformed them into extraordinary lovers of the Lord.

All baptized Christians are called to grow in holiness, to be perfected in the law of Jesus, and to follow in His way. In responding to this call, a new vision takes place as a sparkle of His love glistens in the eyes of the believer. When others see this, they are mysteriously attracted by this eternal quality of goodness. Its "superhuman" power transforms those in pain as they become uplifted, encouraged," and inspired to strive toward goals which make them, by all standards, truly heroic.

As physicians of faith, the needs of your patients must be seen by you and the depth of your Christian vocation must be always seen by them. Like Bartimaeus begging the Lord "to see," [22] we, too, plead for this gift – to see ourselves as we really are and to see with a "faith vision" all who look to us in their need. Above all, we plead for the sparkle of softness in our eyes so that all may see the depth of His divine love. This we ask through Christ our Lord.

---

[22] Mk 10: 46-52

Dedicating Yourself to the Kingdom[1]

Sometimes the modern physician is accused, and rightly so, of "playing God." With "*dis-grace*," human life is taken and then, in an error of "great omnipotence," attempts to create life are sought.

On the other hand, the Catholic physician's work is Christ-centered. Consecrated at baptism as priest, prophet, and king, the work is realized through "*divine grace*." In unity with the Divine Physician, the broken bodies and minds of patients are restored, not for personal gain, but for the glory of the Father.

When Jesus stood before Pilate, He revealed His Kingship was not of this world but He was there "to testify to the truth. Everyone who belongs to the truth listens to my voice."[2] The physician defending truth is rewarded with the crown of Christ the King which, unlike the perishable crown, is eternity.

Today, kings are not a fashionable notion. However, working for possessions and dedicating your life towards its achievement can be a person's "god" or "king." The emphasis of the non-believer whose god is the "dolce vita," may be directed towards attaining pleasure, wealth, power, or honor. The person of faith, however, strives for perfection in following Christ and must make unity with the living God the highest goal.

---

[1] Lorenzetti, Dino (1980) "Message From the Spiritual Advisor," The Linacre Quarterly: Vol. 47: No. 2, Article 2

[2] Jn 18:37

Jesus said, "The kingdom of God is within your midst."[3] An essential truth of Christianity is that Jesus became man and the only real image of God is contained in humanity. Remember, our Lord said, "Amen, I say to you, whatever you did for one of these least brothers of mine, you did for me."[4]

The physician has no problems encountering "the least brothers [sisters]" as they are ever present. When the response is generous in love and action by defending the deprived, healing the sick, and comforting the dying, the physician quickly becomes the recipient of divine grace.

What an extraordinary privilege to represent Christ in all of these experiences! Unlike earthly kings who must rely on their limited resources for power and strength, your heavenly King has the totality of power and He shares it generously with you in His word and the Eucharist. You have the opportunity to bring His strength to an indifferent world by consuming yourself in His mission. With your patients, you have more than a physician-patient relationship. You have the actuality of Christ working in you, healing through your (His) hands and being His personal emissary, assisting our sister and brothers in Christ – to the Kingdom.

---

[3] Lk 17:25
[4] Mt 25:40

The Physician and the Mystical Body of Christ[1]

Through social media, TV, internet, and the advent of cell phones, there is an instant awareness of the mind and heart of people throughout the world. The sports, political, financial, and economic events are transmitted immediately, so that millions, as one world, can witness the happenings of the day and reflect on what they have seen, read, or heard. Likewise, with the exposition of famine, wars, disasters, and sufferings, one can feel the pain as if it were being personally experienced.

The physician, while touching the sick patient, researching new techniques and procedures for healing, or discovering the latest and most effective medications, realizes that the impact of this service goes beyond the individual, for it affects the whole community. St. Paul says, "the body is not one member, but many" and, "God has so constructed the body as to give greater honor to a part that is without it, so that there may be no division in the body, but that the parts may have the same concern for one another. If [one] part suffers, all the parts suffer with it; if one part is honored, all the parts share its joy."[2]

You are in His mystical body and our Lord Jesus sees and "feels" the good you are doing. Your spiritual strength, united with His, is far more powerful in

---

[1] Lorenzetti, Dino (1981) "Message from the Spiritual Advisor," The Linacre Quarterly: Vol. 48: No. 3, Article 2
[2] 1 Cor 12:24-26

affecting new life than a cluster of electronic cells that generate power. Your work is vital. Your will to heal is critical and is combined with your patient's will to be healed. Through your presence, the sick person is infinitely blessed, and in your touch, the patient is touched by the Divine.

St. John speaks of Jesus when he writes, "All things came to be through him, and without him nothing came to be."[3] When you, as a physician of faith, receive Jesus in the Eucharist, you intimately share in that oneness of His mystical body. Every person born, from the beginning of time to the end of time, are also in Him. Therefore, as the Catholic physician performs work in Christ and heals but a single person, all of humanity is affected.

Your good and holy work is like the stone striking still waters which has a ripple effect throughout the pond. So, too, are all the members of His body affected through your dedication and faith in healing the sick. You become instrumental in restoring faith, in strengthening those debilitated, in giving hope to those depressed, and in proclaiming the promise of new life to those facing death.

As your humanity is intermingled in His divinity, you see and touch everyone from the past, those living in the present, and beyond tomorrow. Your vocation affects all of humanity. It affects eternity.

---

[33] Jn 1: 3

As a Priestly Vocation[1]

The physician and priest both possess the two sacred vocations dedicated exclusively toward bringing new life to their brothers and sisters. As disciples of medicine use all gifts given to restore the sick to the fullness of life, they unite themselves with Jesus who declares, "I am the Resurrection and the Life."[2]

Above all, the Christian physician holds a sacrosanct office and thus uplifts the sick (just as the priest does the sinner) to the fullness of health. The medical doctor is blessed with gifts to bridge the "forces of nature" with the ailing patient. Seen as a catalyst, all is exercised and brought to bear, relying on the strength of God's providence and the guidance of the Spirit, to assist the sick in being restored to health.

The physician, as the priest, desires to orchestrate words, love, prayers, and skills so that the sick person will be lifted to the rhythmic harmony of oneness with the Divine. Disorders, then, are relieved, painful groans are raised to cheerful songs and brilliant smiles, and the infirm are resurrected to full humanness.

At the liturgy of the Eucharist, the priest prays, "Lord Jesus Christ, with faith in Your love and mercy I eat Your body and drink Your blood. Let it not bring me

---

[1] Lorenzetti, Dino (1981) "Message from the Spiritual Advisor," The Linacre Quarterly: Vol. 48: No. 1, Article 2 *and* No. 4, Article 2
[2] Jn 11:25

condemnation, but health in mind and body." The physician, as a faithful "priest," in glorifying God, unites all efforts with Jesus. A consecration is experienced, as through the physician's intercession the miracle of God's grace restores the sick to health in mind and body.

In the Lord's name, the priest extends his hands upon the sinner; physicians extend their hands upon the sick so that the fallen are renewed and the weak are strengthened. With caution, they proceed to ensure their actions do not lead them to condemnation. Instead, it is their noblest desire that their prayers and works will strengthen the persons they meet, giving them "newer" life, and thus benefitting them as they journey toward salvation.

In the mystery of loving our brothers and sisters in Christ, in touching the very sacredness of the person, both physician and priest become a part of the promise of new life.

Yours, indeed, is a sacred vocation. It is more than practicing medicine – for a person is more than flesh, just as the Eucharist is more than bread. United with Jesus, you are called to holiness; you have eternity. The sick invite you to pray (to call upon God to help them), to consecrate (to change their illness to health) and resurrect them (to prepare them for a new life). Surely then, you are more than a physician; you are PRIESTLY as well.

Beneficiaries of His Largesse[1]

Very often the beneficiaries of large estates, the recipients of expensive gifts, and individuals awarded important offices are not necessarily those who are most *deserving*, but instead are persons *favored* and *loved* by their benefactor.

Priests' and physicians' commissions were given to them by Christ Himself. He, as the divine benefactor, appointed each of them to heal, to love, and to proclaim His name in their ministry. As the largesse of His gifts is freely and undeservedly given to them, they are, in turn, expected to be dispensed to His people, not begrudgingly, but with joy and peace.

Our Lord Jesus has affirmed, "It was not you who chose me, but I who chose you and appointed you to go and bear fruit that will remain, so that whatever you ask the Father in my name he may give you. This I command you: love one another."[2]

Jesus commands the seed to bear luscious fruit, and He commands us to love, so that as bearers of His grace, those who come to us may be nourished and strengthened on their journey to Him.

In order to bear fruit in abundance, it is necessary that the soil be disposed, that the fertile seed be planted in

---

[1] Lorenzetti, Dino (1982) "Message from the Spiritual Advisor," The Linacre Quarterly: Vol. 49: No. 1, Article 2
[2] Jn 15:16-17

the rich earth, and that there be proper rain and sunshine for the seed to grow and fructify.

Loving physicians are to be disposed to hear the Word of the Lord and respond with generosity to His call. They are to trust in His rain of graces and His sunshine of love and to proceed with confidence to administer the art of healing with the assurance that His Spirit is within them. Then, almost unaware, during the process of ministering to His people, the miracle of His grace occurs. Thus, the name of the Lord is glorified and praised as success is achieved through the works of their hands.

The photographic relays of Voyager I and II, which were launched in 1977, have revealed to us the marvels of the planets, the awesomeness of the galaxy, and the precision of the universe. Both spacecraft probably have enough power left to keep gathering data for us through 2024.[3] Amazing. While these photographic scenes and data are surely extraordinary, they merely portray the ordinary workings of God's creation in what is called, in common parlance, the "natural order."

As in the physical realm, there is also an "order" in the human condition that is ever present. Some scientists, through their experiments, have tried to disprove this but history has repeatedly shown, to the contrary, that there is a rational phenomenon, a reflection of the

---

[3] https://www.space.com/voyager-2-on-its-own-nasa-deep-space-network-upgrades.html

divine wisdom, an expression of love that allows us to be united with God.

This divine wisdom is manifested especially in the work of artists and scientists when achievements of success can be attributed, not to their skills alone, but to the spiritual and motivating force within them which can only be described as a mystery.

Botanists and horticulturists, when speaking of this mystery, refer to it as TLC or "tender loving care" phenomenon. Basically, it is their gentle, God-like attitude toward plant life that has a positive effect on plants. Physicians who lovingly care for their people and treat them beyond a professional manner, extending a loving concern for their needs, also achieve a remarkable record of success: the TLC phenomenon.

For the loving person, the manner in which gifts are given is often more important than the present itself. When selecting a gift for an important occasion, one attempts to choose the right wrapping paper, the matching ribbon and bow, as well as the proper greeting card, so that the gift is not seen as being just "ordinary," but truly special; the loving wrapping/ presentation of the gift.

When gifts of service are wrapped in love, compassion, kindness, and with a prophetic message of hope, they are elevated to our highest expectations in the natural order. Then they become special: they are heart-filled; they are in union with His divine Sacred Heart and the giver becomes an instrument of His redemption.

In being truly human, truly loving, truly gentle, the gifts of service are blessed with a "specialness." They possess a quality of goodness which, when dispensed lovingly to others, becomes easily recognizable. The "secret ingredient" is revealed, namely love, which is the height of perfection in the natural order for humankind. Then, the beauty of our gifts is sanctified. The giver and the receiver are looked upon as favored individuals, for so indeed they are – loved and favored by God. As beneficiaries of the largesse, we are not necessarily deserving, but favored and loved.

The Clown of Godspell[1]

A physician is usually stereotyped as serious, calm, well-dressed, and ready for the handling of the most difficult cases. Quite frequently, this stereotype fits the profession, and yet – may I say this with reverence – perhaps physicians, like priests, should be clowns.

Perhaps you remember the Broadway and movie production of "Godspell" in which the Divine Healer, Jesus, is portrayed as a clown, down to the pom poms on his shoes. When Jesus walked this earth, healing and restoring us to fullness of life, He was criticized, laughed at, and seen as the perfect fool. He was totally misunderstood by the authorities and the multitude; as He gave His all for the very ones He loved, they demeaned His humanness and demanded His death. In spite of this treatment, He continued His journey to do the will of the Father.

The true clown thinks of the other person. As a comic, happiness is sought in the locked soul of the child-like individual. With the simplicity of style, smiles and laughter are provoked to the surface of faces which may be saddened, lonely, or burdened with pain.

The results are the uplifting of the individual, the unloved feel loved, the poor are filled. To be an object of laughter, perhaps a break of protocol, can be judged

---

[1] Lorenzetti, Dino (1985) "Message from the Spiritual Advisor: The Case for Being a Clown," The Linacre Quarterly: Vol. 52: No. 3, Article 2

by observers in different ways. For some, it is nonsense and stupidity, for others it is humility, and for those of faith, it is being Christ-like.

The clown has nothing to say – the clown is judged by action. In "Godspell," there is a prayer in song... "To see thee more clearly, to love thee more dearly, to follow thee more nearly."

How do we see Thee? What is it all about? Oh, to be a clown!

Yes, Lord, I Will Serve[1]

Every physician of faith believing in Jesus, like the apostles, has been called personally by the Lord to "follow Him." The mission is Jesus continuing His own work in and through you, in an ever-deepening communion. It is only as physicians united to Christ that you, like the apostles, can heal the sick and make disciples of all nations.

The call that each has received from the Lord is certainly unexpected, unmerited, and in many ways unique; however, it has compelled a freely-given response from you: "Yes, Lord, I will serve." The vocation, the call, had nothing to do with your culture, finances, temperament, or even experience. The invitation to serve does not presuppose holiness and certainly offers no guarantee that those accepting will not fall at a later date. In fact, it is almost guaranteed that we will fall. However, this response does allow a covenant to be established, and thus a profound bond of unity exists between each individual and Jesus Christ.

When St. Peter "left all" to follow Jesus, leaving his initial investment of a boat and a few nets appeared, at first, to be incidental. Yet his response to leaving "all" ultimately included death and crucifixion; he died professing his faith in Christ. Certainly, Peter "fell" during his walk with Christ, with denials and failures.

---

[1] Lorenzetti, Dino J. (1983) "Message from the Spiritual Advisor," The Linacre Quarterly: Vol. 50: No. 1, Article 2

But, Peter repented, took up his cross, and followed in the Master's footsteps.

Jesus uses the simile of a yoke, or a double harness, to explain His intimate companionship as He journeys with us on our road. When we are yoked with Him, rhythmically walking in the same direction, the "yoke is easy and the burden light."[2] However, should one pull in a different direction and not follow Christ's lead, then a choking sensation is experienced: a struggle, pain, and lack of progress. In our journey through life, following Jesus, having been yoked with Him at Baptism, His spirit strengthens, comforts, and encourages our vocation. Thus, our mission is successful, as it is in tune with His way, truth, and life. We serve, yoked, together.

Yours is a special function in the Body of Christ when you responded, "Yes, Lord, I will serve." Like St. Paul, you "... fill up what is lacking in the suffering of Christ for the sake of His Body, the Church"[3] Jesus has sent the Holy Spirit to inspire, animate, and guide you to carry out the work that only you can accomplish.

---

[2] Mt 11:29-30
[3] Col 1:24

The Mystery of a Vocation[1]

The mystery of pain is the milieu in which the physician works. Associated with pain is a peculiar suffering which signals that the body is undergoing some physical illness. In an attempt to decipher the ailment, the doctor proceeds to use skills to help the patient obtain relief and strive toward recovery.

The doctor is so close to the mystic union of the sufferer that it's difficult to discern why the vocation of medicine was chosen, just as it is impossible for a child to explain why he is playing with a ball. There is a certain magnetism that assures the physician, as well as the child, this is just what has to be done at this time in their lives.

Philippe Petit, a tightrope walker, after being arrested for walking a rope between the World Trade Twin Towers in 1974, was asked why he would attempt such a crazy and dangerous stunt. He replied, "If I see three oranges, I have to juggle. If I see two towers, I have to walk."[2] Sometimes, we are just drawn to a vocation.

The medical profession is involved in a mystery and the patients sent to the physicians are indeed a challenge to their faith. Yet, somehow, these are the very people that will help bring the doctor to salvation.

---

[1] Lorenzetti, Dino J. (1978) "Message From the Spiritual Advisor," The Linacre Quarterly: Vol. 45: No. 1, Article 1
[2] https://www.nydailynews.com/services/new-york-then-now/manhattan/petit-walks-tightrope-twin-towers-1974-article-1.2308431

In the pilgrim journey on the road to holiness, these patients are those whom you — and often you alone — can help. You are their "actual grace." There may be times when your honest complaint is, "Why me?"— perhaps, the same human cry of Jesus at Mt. Olivet: "Father, if you are willing, take this cup away from me." Yet, "still, not my will but yours be done."[3]

There is just a brief distinction between love and violence: between the kiss and the bite, between the touch and the slap, between the delivery and the abortion. There is a difference between the secular and the Catholic, for the Catholic physician is to render services of love — love that heals. As the gift of healing is given, the Lord blesses the doctor, in exchange. So, the joy of gift-giving is a daily experience for the physician of prayer, trusting in the Spirit to guide every action.

The physician's presence is a sign of hope to those in pain. The patient looks upon the doctor, as did the crippled man looking at Peter and John in the temple, hoping for the miracle of grace and to be restored to the fullness of good health.

We thank God for dedicated physicians. You are special people. You touch life, death, and eternity. You are Christ-like persons who heal and do good. We salute you - we respect you - we pray for you. May God always bless you.

---

[3] Lk 22: 42

Section 2: Be Inspired by Scripture

We Are Tenants in the Vineyard[1]

Jesus gives us this parable:

"There was a landowner who planted a vineyard, put a hedge around it, dug a wine press in it, and built a tower. Then he leased it to tenants and went on a journey. When vintage time drew near, he sent his servants to the tenants to obtain his produce. But the tenants seized the servants and one they beat, another they killed, and a third they stoned. Again he sent other servants, more numerous than the first ones, but they treated them in the same way. Finally, he sent his son to them, thinking, 'They will respect my son.' But when the tenants saw the son, they said to one another, 'This is the heir. Come, let us kill him and acquire his inheritance.'"[2]

The tenants in question were entrusted with a commission to care for the vineyard and be accountable to the owner for their efforts. Having been given the privilege to serve, they felt it was their right to usurp. With greed in their hearts, they proceeded to commit

---

[1] Lorenzetti, Dino J. (1977) "Message from the Spiritual Advisor," The Linacre Quarterly: Vol. 44: No. 3, Article 2
[2] Mt 21: 33-38

repeated acts of violence for personal gain, rather than to submit to accountability.

All of us have to account to someone. Among those who have the greatest accountabilities for their professionalism and behavior are physicians, as their office was made possible only through the involvement, encouragement, and expense of a given community. Historically, it was the determined effort of sincere people to construct schools for the training of medical students so that they and their children could benefit from these services. It is, then, through a due process of selection that qualified candidates who value life and the sacredness of the individual are nominated and considered for this high office.

Accountability falls to its lowest level when one has to be compelled to do a job well, otherwise face litigation or disgrace from fellow colleagues, patients, or the community.

The most noble level of accountability is when one performs the challenge of this high office because you "love God with all your heart and your neighbor as yourself."[3] God sees all things and authentic services of healing. The physician proves to be a credit to those people who have given their trust. As a good steward, one uses the gifts God has given and performs to the best of his or her abilities. With our human imperfections, the good works accomplished enrich lives around us as we continue our redemptive mission

---

[3] Mk 12: 30-31

as extensions of Christ. Unlike the unjust steward who needed to manipulate invoices to survive, our accounts are in order and our investments of good works have multiplied a hundredfold.

When the authority of Jesus was challenged, He responded, "...even if you do not believe me, believe the works, so that you may realize that the Father is in me and I am in the Father."[4] In other words, the results speak for themselves.

Since all gifts have been to us, our accountability rests in how they have been shared. For when "I was hungry – thirsty – homeless – sick ..." Jesus said, "Whenever you did this for one of the least important of these brothers of mine, you did it for Me!"[5]

Medical Economics, or investing and using resources wisely, is something known to most physicians. However, the bottom line of the balance sheet, in fine print, is the warning – "What profit would there be for one to gain the whole world and forfeit his life?"[6]

Examination of conscience is difficult and often painful, for in the process, we volunteer to see ourselves just as we are. It is then we rightly pray for God's mercy: for accountability demands a balance between mercy and justice.

---

[4] Jn 10:38
[5] Mt 25:40
[6] Mt 16:26

The Catholic physician believes that God sees all things and nothing goes unnoticed. The good performed is not in *partnership* with the Lord, but in *union* with Him – just as the branch produces fruit only when it's attached to the vine.

And so the physician continues the vocation as a good tenant in the vineyard, working with joy and hope, so that when the journey ends in the vineyard, the voice of God says – "Here is my beloved 'physician' in whom I am well pleased – Come into the kingdom that I have prepared for YOU."

There Are No Small Gestures: Veronica, Simon, & Dismas[1]

At the sixth station in the Way of the Cross, a woman named Veronica is seen wiping the face of Jesus on His agonizing journey to Calvary. Instantly she is rewarded for her act of kindness as Jesus presents her with a true portrait of Himself, even while He is in the depth of great suffering and passion. His bloodstained picture portrays His willingness to suffer for the redemption of all humankind.

The words of Veronica are not recorded but her simple gesture will be remembered for all ages. Her small act of courage and compassion is truly monumental for, in her love, she literally touched Jesus.

When Simon of Cyrene was given the cross of Christ, he didn't realize this Calvary journey was related to all of humankind's redemption. When listening to the jeers, sneers, curses, and insults which were directed at the Christ, he was able to buffet the hurts and uplift the painful cross for the God of love. It is beyond our comprehension, yet true, that "God needed Simon."

Dismas, virtually helpless while nailed to the cross, was fearless in his defense of Jesus as he loudly declared, "This man has done nothing wrong." Jesus

---

[1] Edited from Lorenzetti, Dino J. (1986) "Message from the Spiritual Advisor: Small Actions...Great Rewards," The Linacre Quarterly: Vol.53: No.3, Article 1 *and* (1984) Symbols in Many Forms, Vol.51: No.1, Article 2

immediately declared him a saint: "Amen, I say to you, today you will be with me in Paradise."[2]

Small actions? Great rewards! Jesus is never outdone in generosity. When it comes to offering hospitality, Jesus reminds us: "Whoever receives you [your patients] receives me, and whoever receives me receives the one who sent me."[3] Receive your patients as Christ.

Doctors, I see you as the Simon, Veronica, and Dismas of today. God needs you. You are nearest to Jesus in the sick you serve, in the care you give them, in the cross you carry for them. Your actions and your response, when performed in love, may seem like small gestures. Yet in the eyes of the Lord, they are great signs of your faith.

See in your patient, veiled in human flesh, the suffering Christ before you; you have encountered the Savior. When your days on this earth are completed, may you who have touched Christ, carried His cross, and defended His life, hear His loving words of welcome to the Kingdom: WELCOME, my good and faithful servant, for "today you will be with Me in Paradise."

---

[2] Lk 23: 41-43
[3] Mt 10: 40

Physicians as Innkeepers[1]

St. Luke, in the gospel narrative on the birth of Jesus, speaks of an innkeeper in Bethlehem who refused hospitability to Mary and Joseph when they applied for lodging, stating that he had "no room for them."[2]

Perhaps if the innkeeper knew who these strangers were who were asking for accommodations, he would have attempted some type of arrangement. It is obvious he was unaware of the Messiah veiled before him in the womb of Mary.

Physicians, to some extent, are "innkeepers" who are in a special position to welcome (or refuse) into their offices or hospitals those needing healing: the sick, the confused, and the injured. Some patients are reluctant to call a doctor's office as they fear the receptionist will say, "Sorry, the doctor is not scheduling any new appointments." In other words, "There is no room for you."

When the Good Samaritan brought the victim beaten among robbers to the inn, he had no qualms showing compassion to this stranger. In fact, he was so magnanimous in his generosity that his example epitomizes the loving of one's neighbor.

Our society is overcrowded with people yearning for acceptance, to be welcomed, to be healed. Depression

---

[1] Catholic Physicians' Guild (1984) "Message from the Spiritual Advisor," The Linacre Quarterly: Vol. 51: No. 2, Article 2
[2] Lk 2: 7

is still one of the greatest ills of our time. How blessed is the physician who sees this vocation as hosting the sick, rejected, poor, and noninfluential.

The innkeeper in Bethlehem was likely a good person and we cannot be harsh with him. When he was unable to oblige them, he could have been the very individual who referred Joseph and Mary "up the road" to the cave.

Likewise, no one wants to be harsh with a physician who unintentionally overlooks the opportunity to do good for another. However, as a people of faith, we are all called to be sensitive to the presence of Christ hidden in all who call for our services. It is important that, at all times, we be gracious to the stranger who allows us to witness the great commandment in our faith: love our neighbor as ourselves.

The physician's attitude, tone of voice, compassion, service, and dedication are all encompassed with generosity in loving care to those who call. The physician of faith treats all patients as sacred persons, created in the image of the Creator, and destined for eternal life. Concern is beyond the science of medicine: it is rooted in love.

On Being a Prudent and Vigilant Bridesmaid Awaiting the King[1]

Jesus told a parable of a wedding feast where ten bridesmaids awaited the coming of the groom.[2] He explained that only half, or five of the ten bridesmaids, had prepared themselves with sufficient oil to keep their lamps burning in readiness for his arrival. These bridesmaids were called sensible, or the prudent ones.

From time immemorial, the Church has been understood to be the "bride" of Christ. All who are baptized in the Church, both male and female, are "brides" of Christ. Thus, the "wise bridesmaids" of the scriptures are those individuals who are always prudently awake, preparing for His coming, looking forward to the glorious union with Christ.

As Catholic physicians, you are among those prudent bridesmaids who are vigilant, who have invested your energies not on perishable vanities, but on values that are lasting, namely the eternal kingdom. Jesus spoke of the values which constitute His kingdom: feeding the poor (with food, knowledge and the necessities of life), caring for the sick (those in need of healing, both of mind and body), visiting the prisoner (the depressed, the drug addict, the shut-in, the unloved), clothing the naked (with garments of dignity, hope, and the

---

[1] Lorenzetti, Dino (1982) "Message from the Spiritual Advisor," The Linacre Quarterly: Vol. 49: No. 2, Article 2
[2] Mt 25

security of their civil rights) and above all, treating the whole person with love.

Unfortunately, some physicians, like the foolish bridesmaids, are not alert. They have fallen asleep and are not ready for the call that "the groom has arrived." Tendencies toward apathy, greed, sinful pride, or having developed a hardness of heart can lead to lethargic behaviors (their lanterns are extinguished – burned out in futility) and they are spiritually unprepared for the coming of the Lord.

In the eucharistic liturgy, the Church proclaims the mystery of faith with the acclamation: "Christ has died, Christ is risen, *Christ will come again.*" In baptism we are sealed with the oil of salvation, prudently awaiting His coming, our Risen Savior. There is no time to delay, but immediately we must prepare to become more compassionate, forgiving, and generous – voicing protests against harmful legislation to our brothers and sisters and, above all, witnessing Christ to His kingly people.

Your talents generously given become kingly gifts and will endure forever. Since you are truly "churched" as His bride, you will be welcomed by Christ Himself, your groom, to share at His royal banquet prepared for those – yes, you – who love Him.

Physician as Shepherd: Psalm 23[1]

Skilled craftsmen universally have captured the scriptural image of Christ, the Good Shepherd, in their works of art. They portray the loving, compassionate Lord Jesus with His rod and staff, surrounded by the sheep awaiting His next move. This theme of Psalm 23 is applied to both bishops and priests in their evangelical apostolate. Could the physician be cited as a shepherd also?

> "The Lord is my shepherd; there is nothing I lack. In green pastures he makes me lie down; to still waters he leads me; he restores my soul. He guides me along right paths for the sake of his name. Even though I walk through the valley of the shadow of death, I will fear no evil, for you are with me; your rod and your staff comfort me.
>
> You set a table before me in front of my enemies; You anoint my head with oil; my cup overflows. Indeed, goodness and mercy will pursue me all the days of my life; I will dwell in the house of the Lord for endless days."[2]

---

[1] Edited from Catholic Physicians' Guild (1977) "Message From the Spiritual Advisor," The Linacre Quarterly: Vol. 44: No. 2, Article 7 *and* Lorenzetti, Dino (1985) "Message from the Spiritual Advisor: Image of the Good Shepherd," The Linacre Quarterly: Vol. 52: No. 4, Article 2

[2] Ps 23

In our highly technological society, agricultural scenes of sheep and shepherds are hardly compatible with busy cities, speedy ambulances and ultra-modern hospitals. Therefore, one can readily ask, is the metaphor of shepherd and sheep relevant today?

The physician's responsibility to leave those who are healthy and care for the sick, abandoned, confused, diseased, and weak is indisputable. The choice to give time and life to bring patients toward health surely mirrors Him who lifts His sheep, lost and afraid, onto His shoulders. The patient looks upon the good shepherd to lead the way through the dark valley of illness or disorder, to be guided by the doctor's rod and staff (medical tools) to receive healing with the oils of comfort, and to be loved with the "cup that overflows."

With great confidence in the voice of the shepherd, the vulnerable patient listens carefully to the instructions while trusting and traveling through the dangerous narrow path on the road to recovery.

The Christian physician rejoices as this vocation is re-affirmed and embodies the Good Shepherd. For the doctor knows that only "goodness and mercy will pursue me all the days of my life; I will dwell in the house of the Lord for endless days."[3]

---

[3] Ibid

Observing Mary[1]

A beautiful mark of distinction between the Catholic physician and physicians, in general, is the former's devotion to Mary, the Mother of God. St. Luke, the evangelist and physician, was among the first writers to record in sacred scriptures the events of salvation history concerning Mary, our Mother.

Since that time, there is hardly a hamlet in the world which does not have a church named in her honor as well as a large number of children christened with her name. Mary's loyalty, obedience, and love of God are constantly presented as a model for all of us to follow. Her life of prayer and dedication pleased the Lord as she lived her special vocation in faith.

The Catholic physician is appreciative of women: she offers the habitat of her very being for the continuation of life and of her closeness to the divine. Acknowledging her labor and delivery, her pain and recovery, the doctor perceives the specialness in her person. She certainly has an uplifted dignity as God chose woman as a means for His only Son's entry into this world.

Mothers renew their consciousness of "bonding," that is, that intimate relationship they have with their children, often developed in a mystical way through nursing, affection, and lovingly gazing face-to-face

---

[1] Lorenzetti, Dino J. (1979) "Message from the Spiritual Advisor," The Linacre Quarterly: Vol. 46: No. 3, Article 2

with their babies. This "oneness," perfected by Mary with her Son, can be imitated by the physician, as well. Modeling Mary and mothers, the doctor transmits solace, comfort, and strength through touching, healing, praying, and sharing face-to-face with patients in need.

Logic and science express theories, but not complete or satisfactory explanations, on the mystery of humankind and the universe. Humanity is not simply explained with science as we are intrigued with the divine. No one's life has ever been more intrigued with the Trinity than Mary and, just as St. Luke observed, physicians would do well to examine her for a more complete understanding of humanity. It is well to note that her obedience to God brought about life. Her faith became the vehicle to see her Son as we witnessed miracles take place: wine from water, health from sickness, salvation from sin.

Is the Catholic doctor different from other doctors? If devoted to Mary, the answer is certainly "yes." There is a hidden strength that has never been known to fail. "Never was it known that anyone who fled to thy protection, implored thy help, or sought thy intercession was left unaided."[2] Don't underestimate Catholic physicians: they have good connections.

---

[2] Memorare prayer to Mary

Sirach Extols the Physician[1]

In the book of Sirach, the author praises the vocation of the physician:

> "Make friends with the doctor, for he is essential to you; God has also established him in his profession. From God the doctor has wisdom... Then give the doctor his place lest he leave; you need him too, for there are times when recovery is in his hands. He too prays to God that his diagnosis may be correct and his treatment bring about a cure."[2]

The most distinguishing factor between a doctor of faith and a nonbelieving colleague is that the former is always aware that God plays the most important role in the sacred work of healing. Privileged to explore the wonder and beauty of the human body and mind with the skill and art of medicine, the believing physician treats patients with science, but with great humility. The physician is but the instrument of the Almighty.

As a Eucharistic member of the Church, faith-filled and in sacramental union with Jesus, you, the physician, become one with Christ. The sick perceive in you the presence of the Lord as you speak, touch, and care for them. They envision the divine gifts

---

[1] Lorenzetti, Dino J. (1988) "Message From the Spiritual Advisor," The Linacre Quarterly: Vol. 55: No. 2, Article 2
[2] Sir 38: 1-2, 12-14

flowing in the services you render in love. While these results cannot be tabulated through objective or scientific criteria, their effects are well seen and felt by those blessed in faith.

Love mandates going beyond what is expected in one's work. It exceeds law and protocol; it is total giving. This is the Christian principle which is contrary to a society prone to "count the cost" or "study the data." Love is the call of all but, in a special way, to those in health care services.

When Jesus dined at the house of Simon the Pharisee, a "sinful" woman who "crashed the party" demonstrated her faith as she washed His feet with her tears, wiped them with her hair, and perfumed them with oil. Certainly her behavior was beyond customary hospitality. In response for her generous love, Jesus declared that not only were her sins forgiven, but that her faith was her salvation.[3]

A physician of faith is filled with hope and trusts in the power of the Divine Healer. As Sirach advocates: "Pray to God that [your] diagnosis may be correct and [your] treatment bring about a cure." Strengthened with the grace of the Spirit, you witness the Gospel through your vocation. The joy of your services certainly exceeds monetary gain or fame, as Christ promises that sins will be forgiven and you, too, will be a welcome candidate to the Kingdom.

---

[3] Lk 7: 36-50

Section 3: Practicing the Practice

Fasting and Praying Before Practice[1]

In the study of iconography, artists acknowledge that they spend considerable time in prayer, fasting, and reflection before they attempt to paint an icon. They interpret their work not only as a piece of art but also as a sacred image which is seen as an object for veneration.

The artists in the Middle Ages viewed their masterpieces as creations from their deep relationship with their Creator. These masterful works have in the past, and for generations to come, served their purpose in bringing humankind to loftier heights and to a spiritual enrichment.

While spirited artists touch earthly materials so that they may become awesome delights of art, physicians, with their spirit of healing, touch and uplift patients who are destined for eternity.

Charismatic healers acknowledge, in preparation for a prayer service, they fast and pray so the Spirit of the Lord will work through them and the sick may be healed and the Father glorified.

The Scriptures record many incidents in which Jesus fasted throughout His public life, and also instructed

---

[1] Lorenzetti, Dino (1985) "Message from the Spiritual Advisor: God Influences Professions," The Linacre Quarterly: Vol. 52: No. 1, Article 2

His Apostles that certain kinds of healing can be obtained only through prayer and fasting.

The traditional teaching of the Church is for the priest to fast before he celebrates Holy Mass and the faithful are also obliged to fast prior to the reception of the Eucharist.

All physicians are aware of the science of medicine but few are familiar with the spiritual gifts which are afforded to those who unite themselves with the Spirit of the Lord before exercising their vocation.

It should be tried.

Before undertaking serious action, surgery, or commencing treatment on a patient where the miracle of God's grace is called upon for success, fast and pray. Unite yourself with the Spirit of the Lord, so that you recreate His masterpiece. By your touching of the sick, may your "artistic icon" be a radiant object for veneration, so that God will be praised as His people see the sick person gain inner strength. In the raising of "your Lazarus" to new life, you show yourself as being more than a physician – you are an instrument of God.

Seeking Solutions Through Petition[1]

Scientists throughout the world are to be commended for their untiring efforts and for their great successes in searching for solutions to help those suffering from illnesses which are devastating to all humankind.

In the 1980s, AIDS caused great concern and fear in our society and continues to be a challenge. Today, pandemics, malignant cancer, obesity, and heart disease are top medical priorities. While humanity desperately looks to medical research for successful solutions for these devastating diseases, the words of Jesus Christ should be taken seriously: "Ask and it will be given to you; seek and you will find; knock and the door will be opened to you."[2]

The answers to these perplexing problems are presently locked behind the "closed door." Our Divine Lord has instructed us to "ask." Should we not, as a people of faith, dedicate ourselves to prayer, begging for His grace?

Should we not plead for His spirit of wisdom, counsel, and understanding to descend upon those scientists dedicated to medical research? Should we not "seek" for a philosophy of life which will enhance His people rather than debase them? To teach love, self-restraint,

---

[1] Lorenzetti, Dino J. (1987) "Message from the Spiritual Advisor: The Search for Solutions," The Linacre Quarterly: Vol. 54: No. 4, Article 1
[2] Mt 7: 7

to conform to the laws of nature, and to promote a way of life in which the Son of God is revered, rather than the gods of men?

What a beautiful new day it will be when there is an "open sesame." The locked door is opened and rays of sunshine rush in. The polluted waters become fresh again, and the poisoned earth renewed, so that delicious fruits come forth as in the Garden of Eden before the fall of man. Utopia becomes a reality when a sick society begs for forgiveness and is uplifted in His grace.

It is like a good confession. Sins are absolved, the sinner is restored to God's grace and is sent off in peace to sin no more and to bear fruit.

Is this but a dream? In the hearts of those who truly believe, it is possible. Through repetitive knocks through prayer, the door will be opened, the world enlightened, humankind healed: we are forgiven.

Remedies for the deadly diseases, as well as for physical and emotional illnesses, can be found and God's people can rejoice in His peace. How can this be done? Jesus gave us the answer, "Ask and you will receive." This is His promise.

Protecting Yourself From Anxiety[1]

Overwhelmed by technological advances and vast studies which are daily surfaced at computer speed, the physician finds it daunting to keep up with the latest of scientific findings. Physicians are often pressured for better quality medical care and asked some mighty difficult questions.

In a society that yearns for "more," we are faced with the fact that little time remains to enjoy life and to do things important to restore balance. The doctor is in a "catch 22": filled with frustrations and daily rushing to catch up, and yet experiencing a life which is speedily passing by. Unlike other friends or peers, the physician finds it difficult to reflect and enjoy life.

Conscious of the importance of patients needing rest, relaxation, and recreation, the physician must also STOP. Please consider this Psalm:

> "Our life ebbs away under your wrath; our years end like a sigh. Seventy is the sum of our years, or eighty, if we are strong; Most of them are toil and sorrow; they pass quickly, and we are gone...Teach us to count our days aright, that we may gain wisdom of heart... May the favor of the Lord our God be ours. Prosper the work of our hands!"[2]

---

[1] Lorenzetti, Dino J. (1979) "Message From the Spiritual Advisor," The Linacre Quarterly: Vol. 46: No. 1, Article 1
[2] Psalm 90: 9-17

The Catholic physician, continuing the mission of Jesus in healing the sick, must, like Jesus, take time to get away, to pray, to rebalance life.

At every liturgy of the Eucharist, we plead: "In your mercy keep us free from sin and PROTECT US FROM ALL ANXIETY as we wait in joyful hope for the coming of our Savior, Jesus Christ." The person who is protected from all anxieties has found the peace for which the world is searching: those moments of being with Christ, meditating on His teachings, and being healed with His love.

Granted, there is much to do.

And yet, St. Luke warns us with the words of Jesus:

> "Therefore I tell you, do not worry about your life and what you will eat, or about your body and what you will wear. For life is more than food and the body more than clothing... Can any of you by worrying add a moment to your life-span? If even the smallest things are beyond your control, why are you **anxious** [emphasis added] about the rest?"[3]

Your Father knows well what you need. Therefore, relax and "set your heart on His kingdom." Then everything makes sense. Your life is successful; you are at peace; there is hope, for you are awaiting the coming of Our Lord Jesus Christ.

---

[3] Lk 12: 22-26

Fatigue[1]

Tiredness is a way of life for active physicians. While dispensing "relief" medication to patients, aches and pains are a reality known only to themselves. This is part of the sacrifice they endure, standing long hours, and often under great stress, performing intricate procedures.

While the doctor is pressured with frustration, anxieties, and disappointments, time is found to encourage patients afflicted with disorders and diseases. Sometimes it seems as if every "drop" of energy has been drained from the mortal body.

The TV dramas and the movies portray the physician with unlimited vitality, yet the truth of the matter is that even though there is zeal and passion under ordinary circumstances, when tiredness sets in, life undergoes a torturous struggle that is indefinable.

To see real meaning in this vocation, let's turn to the word "sacrifice" as interpreted coming from the word "sacred." Commitment is being united to Jesus, the "perfect sacrifice." All that is given, consummation of self, is done willingly for the good of the people of God. Total giving is a crucifixion for the continuing salvation of humankind. The doctor is in union with Jesus as a special person in the Mystical Body, as the mystery of redemption unfolds.

---

[1] Lorenzetti, Dino (1981) "Message from the Spiritual Advisor," The Linacre Quarterly: Vol. 48: No. 2, Article 3

In the dying process, the pain, the loss, the "wearing out" of oneself has meaning. If it is seen in the dimension of faith, Christianity has purpose, sacrifice has redemption and healing, and the consummation of one's life, like the consummation of salt, gives enrichment to that which it touches. Believing in Jesus, one is forgiven and healed, one is united in suffering, one is raised up beyond the grave, and one has life that is eternal.

Among the last seven words of Jesus on the Cross was, "It is consummated."[2] Worn out, having given all, "He emptied Himself," and within a matter of days, total giving was transformed to the glory of His resurrection.

Jesus preached that all who are weary should come to Him and He would refresh them. The "living water," the source of all life, is Jesus. United with the saving Lord, the physician who "eats [His] flesh and drinks [His] blood"[3] knows, from Jesus' own words, that He abides within. This is where the reservoir of grace can be found. One can tap this well of living water that goes far beyond natural resources of energy, vitamins, or synthetic drugs. Here is the fountain of youth, new life, and renewed strength which can be had for the asking.

---

[2] Jn 19: 30. A more common translations is: "It is finished."
[3] Jn 6: 53

Happiness Is...[1]

The yellow round face with a black-lined crescent mouth and oval filled-in eyes seems to have received the unofficial symbol of what "Happiness is." This non-copyrighted logo is frequently seen with a word or phrase following the quotation to describe what the promoter believes is the highest degree of joy. It may vary from an inexpensive popular beverage to a relaxing vacation on an exotic island. However, to the patient, happiness is going home from the hospital, completely recovered, relieved of pain, returned to life.

A truly happy (blessed) person is one who is in pursuit of eternal life. Motivation and drive are not toward the perishable goods of this life which will vanish, but a willingness to endure even hardships for the kingdom of God which will last forever.

When Jesus began His public ministry in Galilee, He proclaimed eight beatitudes. After His resurrection, He added a ninth when appearing to His apostles in the upper room. He approached the unbelieving Thomas and said, "Have you come to believe because you have seen me? Blessed [happy] are those who have not seen and have believed."[2]

With faith, a physician becomes endowed with a gift of seeing the mysterious regions of the divine. Hope is

---

[1] Lorenzetti, Dino J. (1987) "Message from the Spiritual Advisor: What Happiness Is!" The Linacre Quarterly: Vol. 54: No. 1, Article 1
[2] Jn 20: 29

offered to patients which is intertwined with the promise of the Savior. The physician's love and concern uplift the medical profession to the highest of vocations as its mission unites with the Divine Healer. Oneness with Christ enables the physician to share in the restoration of the patient's health.

What extraordinary joy the patient experiences when encountering the physician who is blessed.

Sometimes along life's journey, we meet a special person who just seems to light up our life with joy: a person who helps us to really see the beauty of the world, the good in others, and the good in ourselves. We often find ourselves amazed at how lucky we were to find such a person, but of course it isn't luck – it is a blessing from God.

We are all called to bring this light and joy of Christ into each other's lives: a physician to the patient. St. Peter puts it in these words: "Although you have not seen him you love him; even though you do not see him now yet believe in him, you rejoice with an indescribable and glorious joy, as you attain the goal of [your] faith, the salvation of your souls."[3]

Dear Doctor – your faith in the invisible God makes you a blessed person indeed, as you see Him in those whom you serve. Yes, happiness is... "blind" faith in Jesus Christ.

---

[3] 1 Peter 1: 8-9

Physician, You Are Healed[1]

Many doctors hear the words of Jesus, "Physician, heal yourself"[2] echoing in their ears when they are faced with personal problems of poor health.

This disturbing statement challenges the person of faith to realize Jesus is inviting His medical emissary on earth to be healed so as to better serve His people in need.

When Simon Peter's mother-in-law was afflicted with a fever, Jesus healed her "...then the fever left her and she waited on them."[3] The words to note are that she immediately served after she was healed.

One's frail human body is often heavily burdened with varied illnesses, worries, fears, and insecurities. The individual feels so weak that it appears all energies are dissipated and therefore one is literally unable to serve.

Physicians, conscious of this reality, should find comfort in the fact that the same healing power Jesus exercised with Peter's mother-in-law is also theirs. Their vocation, when united with Jesus, becomes perfected as they acknowledge their weakness, their sinful state, their total trust in His amazing grace. In doing so, the omnipotent and loving God relieves the

---

[1] Lorenzetti, Dino J. (1988) "Message From the Spiritual Advisor," The Linacre Quarterly: Vol. 55: No. 3, Article 1
[2] Lk 4: 23
[3] Mk 1: 29-31

yoke which is seemingly so oppressive and raises the spirit to new life. "I will put my spirit in you that you may come to life."[4]

At the liturgy of the Mass, before the reception of the Eucharist, the worshipper humbly prays, "Lord, I am not worthy that you should enter under my roof. Only say the Word and I shall be healed."

In the mystery, through God's grace, as this happens, "Physician, you are healed."

---

[4] Ez 37: 14

Searching for the Holy: For You[1]

In the search for a place to be restored to the fullness of health, the sick are motivated to travel long distances, far away from their own homes, to be healed. They are anxious to find an atmosphere of sanctity, to beg for the miracle of healing. Some travel to Lourdes, Fatima, or Jerusalem, just to be at a holy place. The greater number, however, walk to their local church and sit in the awesomeness of holiness to present their petitions.

The desire to meet a sacred person is even more impelling than finding a sacred place. This is evident throughout history, when people crowded around the feet of philosophers, prophets, and saints to listen attentively to their words of wisdom. Vast numbers of people assembled just to be within sight of someone whom they considered to be holy, such as Mother Teresa of Kolkata or Pope John Paul II. Today, the throng gathers for His Holiness, Pope Francis.

In the public ministry of Jesus, great crowds surrounded Him wherever He went. They were looking not only for answers to the mystery of the universe and its Creator, but also for daily food, restoration to health, and for knowledge to free them from their bondage.

---

[1] Lorenzetti, Dino (1982) "Message from the Spiritual Advisor," The Linacre Quarterly: Vol. 49: No. 4, Article 2

St. Matthew tells this story:

> "A woman suffering hemorrhages for twelve years came up behind [Jesus] and touched the tassel on his cloak. She said to herself, 'If only I can touch his cloak, I shall be cured.' Jesus turned around and saw her, and said, 'Courage, daughter! Your faith has saved you.' And from that hour the woman was cured."[2]

"Courage" is the first word Jesus uttered before proceeding to cure the woman. In our modern society, discouragement is a common symptom among the majority of persons who are sick. They need to be encouraged, put at ease, especially before and after surgery, and to be continually uplifted from their discomforts and troublesome ailments.

Your words of encouragement imbued with faith, when given truthfully, prayerfully and in a heartfelt manner, have a tremendous effect on your patient. By God's grace, you are indeed a sacred person. People are anxious to "hang on" to you, to touch the hem of your clothing, for you are able to dispel their fears. Your patients have great faith in you. Their prayers are that they be the recipient of the very healing power hidden within you. Yes, you are that holy person.

---

[2] Mt 9:20-22

Discouragement with Patients[1]

Perhaps one of the greatest temptations the modern physician faces in practice is discouragement. If you "give in" to it, you may find yourself in a state of depression, losing enthusiasm, zeal, and dedication to your work.

With the increasing costs of insurance and the threat of being sued for malpractice, the physician is obliged to practice the profession defensively to avoid any possibility of legal contestation. Often in counseling patients, the doctor is challenged by articles published in popular periodicals which compel the defense of the treatment recommended. In a form of surrender, one is tempted to cater to the wishes of the patient, even if it is not the preferred treatment.

It is in this setting that a doctor might feel, "I've had it," or, "Who needs it?" or "Let someone else carry on. I've done my job." While all of this may be pragmatically logical, still it is not the way Christ works through us.

The physician, like Christ the Savior, accepts not only the centurion (who has total faith)[2] but also the man born blind (who is demanding)[3], the thief on the cross (who is in pain)[4], the woman hemorrhaging (who is

---

[1] Lorenzetti, Dino J. (1983) "Message from the Spiritual Advisor," The Linacre Quarterly: Vol. 50: No. 2, Article 2
[2] Mt 8: 5-13
[3] Mk 10: 46-52
[4] Lk 23: 39-43

[75]

anxious)[5], Mary Magdalene (who was possessed of evil spirits)[6], the woman at the well (an inquirer)[7], St. Thomas (a challenger)[8], St. Peter (who denies Christ)[9], and Nicodemus (the teacher, who is "ignorant").[10]

Through their encounters with Christ – like your patients' contact with you – the weak become strong, and the impossible become possible. You uplift the depressed and paradoxically you are likewise "saved." Your vocation has meaning, you are uplifted from your depression, you become enthusiastic, and your life has activity. United with Jesus who performs the healing, you are His selected loved one through whom His Spirit flows.

All types of patients come to you, those who are anxious, uninformed, fearful, demanding, and above all, challenging. It is through you, the Catholic doctor of faith who, like Christ, lovingly cares that your patients are able to have a change of heart, sinners are able to become saints, and the unholy are able to become whole.

---

[5] Lk 8: 40-48
[6] Lk 8: 2
[7] Jn 4: 4-29
[8] Jn 20: 24-29
[9] Jn 18: 15-27
[10] Jn 3: 1-21

The Redemptive Physician/Patient Relationship[1]

Almost inevitably the patient is the one who searches out the physician. After being troubled with an illness, he or she usually decides that a way must be found to solve the problem. Looking into the professional health care field for a competent physician, the patient decides that you are the one to follow.

Jesus said: "I am the way, the truth and the life,"[2] and, as Christ's hands on earth, the physician is called upon to outline a plan for the patient who needs to be put on the "road to recovery." Even though the path you outline may be difficult, the patient is asking you to chart the way.

Since your patient trusts in you, you are compelled to share the truth. You speak with authority. When a patient is suffering with a terminal illness, it can be most difficult, yet the truth must be told with a gentle tone, with words of hope and faith.

Through the way and truth, you are able to speak of life – new life which continues beyond human suffering and pain.

This patient, once unknown, has now become a very important "partner" in your relationship. He has entrusted his very life into your hands, and with your

---

[1] Lorenzetti, Dino (1984) "Message from the Spiritual Advisor: Physician-Patient Relationship," The Linacre Quarterly: Vol. 51: No. 4, Article 2
[2] Jn 14: 6

treatment, a bond has been established. It has become a relationship with a special status, that is sacred.

Relationships vary with different people. With God, our relationship is absolute: "I will take you as my own people, and I will be your God."[3] Other relationships, as in marriage or in religious life, are solemn. Still others are seen as holy, such as that between physician and patient. In each relationship, there is a commitment to help the other to spiritual happiness and to holiness. For the sick person, you have become a sign of hope.

In this bonding, you have established yourself in a redemptive relationship which is eternal. It is indeed a paradox: a sick, weakened person searches you out to "show the way," and by your actions, "the way is shown to you." A miracle occurs, a change takes place, there is a healing; but this time it takes place in you. You have become the beneficiary of your patient's redemptive suffering.

It is common knowledge that partnerships dissolve at the death of one of the parties. Yet your physician-patient relationship, which is truly sacred, continues into eternity when your partner, your patient, is face-to-face with the Redeemer.

---

[33] Ex 6: 7

We Are Created in the Image of God[1]

When God made humanity to His image and likeness, He gave us life. He actually gave us Himself. The author of the book of Genesis says, "God created mankind in his image; in the image of God he created them; male and female he created them."[2]

When the computer was invented, it was given information and hardware, it was not given life, therefore the computer is not made in the image and likeness of humanity. The computer is able to supply accurate, speedy, and detailed information, but it does not have life (the image of God) to translate that data into the language of *love*.

The loving physician sees patients made in God's image and can apply God-given human talents so that the way to new life can be shown. With professional competence in medicine, the Holy Spirit is relied upon for His sevenfold gifts: wisdom, counsel, understanding, fortitude, knowledge, piety and fear of the Lord, so that patients will be the beneficiaries of the divine assistance.

When Jesus manifested the image of God, He stripped Himself of His glory and became human, showing the way to portray the image of God and to witness His

---

[1] Lorenzetti, Dino (1985) "Message from the Spiritual Advisor: Man in God's Image," The Linacre Quarterly: Vol. 52: No. 2, Article 2
[2] Gen 1:27

presence among His own people. Jesus tells us, "The Father is in me and I in the Father."[3]

As the divine physician, Jesus performed miracles which His humanness, alone, would have been unable to accomplish. The image of God was seen in the healing of the sick, dispelling demons, and raising the dead to life. To show us the way, Jesus prayed, forgave, and at all times was generous to all He encountered. His example taught us that it is in faith that we praise the unseen God by performing acts of love to those whom we do see.

The most undesirable individuals in the respectable society of Jesus' time were the beggars, lepers, prostitutes, thieves, and the alien. It was specifically among these that He performed His apostolic mission, showing them love and concern, uplifting them, accepting them, and inspiring them.

As Christ remains in us through the gift of Baptism, His presence and power continue through our ministry. Thus, in keeping the commandments, we become closer and more perfect in relation to the Father and mysteriously radiate His image.

As the physician of faith witnesses Christ, the image and likeness of God is radiated. When this occurs, the world sees love, hope, peace, and salvation being renewed as the invisible Jesus is seen in the visible physician.

---

[3] Jn 10:38

Section 4: Suffering and Healing

Jesus Experienced Death[1]

Perhaps the most difficult human experience a physician faces is to tell a patient that science can no longer help towards recovery and that death is imminent. Even with the greatest of tact, the practitioner of medicine endures heartfelt pain as this saddening news is revealed to the person who is sick, especially if it happens to be a loved one.

At times, in really not knowing what to say, the physician may apt to remark, "I understand what you are going through." While that may be partially true, the fact is that the doctor really doesn't know what it's like – the anguish, worry, or suffering the patient endures at this particular moment in time.

The Old Testament reports that Moses conversed with Almighty God on different occasions as he led the chosen people to the promised land. Throughout the forty years in the desert, the Israelites constantly complained, even though God performed miracles before their very eyes: feeding them with manna and quail, satisfying their thirst with fresh drinking water, curing their ills, guiding them by day with a column of smoke and at night with a column of fire. God told Moses the Israelites were a "stiff necked people"[2] because they violated God's command for true worship and the people entrusted to Moses were ungrateful and

---

[1] Lorenzetti, Dino J. (1974) "A Catholic Physician - A Person of Faith," The Linacre Quarterly: Vol. 41: No. 4, Article 2
[2] Ex 33:5

difficult. In reading this biblical account, it is not difficult to imagine Moses thinking, "God, there You are in Your comfortable heaven away from it all – really, You don't know what it's like."

On the first Christmas day, in the town of Bethlehem, God settled the question once and for all. In essence He said, "Yes, I do know what it's like – to be human. To love, to live, be rejected, be spit upon, be nailed to a cross, and to die. But I also want you to know something else – there is a life beyond that moment of death and the world will see that suffering has purpose, it's allied with redemption."

What is the response to the question – who is Christ? The general catechetical or theological answer is one that is heard often; namely, He is the Incarnate Word, the Second Person of the Blessed Trinity, the Son of God, the Messiah. Yet the question must be personalized as it was to Peter. "Who do you say that I am?" If we truly believe and are able to transmit this truth to the patient, then the transition from earthly death to heavenly life becomes an acceptable reality for the person of faith. Yes, God knows what it's like. He comforts and consoles, but above all He understands.

Violence and the Author of Life[1]

The Catholic physician today is in a position of unique importance unsurpassed in many years. In a society so imbued with the culture of death, the way must be led in opposition to this philosophy which so violates the ideals of the healing vocation.

Violence resulting in death has become the popular theme for recreation in movies, videogames, and television; it is the technique applied in the abortion clinic; it is employed for "security reasons" in military expediency, and is used as a means of personal gain on the streets of most large cities. Latter incidents can be verified in the daily news reports of break-ins, muggings, and stabbing of innocent citizens who have become pawns and victims. In the larger cities of this country, crimes are recorded as often as once every eighteen minutes.

Physicians bear witness to all of this daily in the emergency rooms of the hospitals they serve.

There has been considerable publicity advocating euthanasia. In some of the public's mind, it is equivalent to "mercy killing" – that is, the direct killing of an individual patient for some "good" reason. One of the standard reasons is to prevent pain and suffering.

The physician – gifted to heal, offer comfort, show compassion always to those in need – would be shocked

---

[1] Catholic Physicians' Guild (1975) "Moderator's Page," The Linacre Quarterly: Vol. 42: No. 2, Article 2

at the action of a physician who would directly kill a patient, even at the patient's request. Medical training is directed at supporting life, not toward the use of any means to directly extinguish it. The role is that of healer, not executioner; success is in curing, not in killing.

In showing compassion for those who are suffering, all physicians — but particularly the Catholic physician — should see patients as their brothers and sisters. The physician treats each person with great care and concern, always mindful of the worth of each individual human life.

Through faith, the Catholic physician knows God as the Author of Life and, as such, the one who reserves the sole right over life. What more noble service could be rendered than to assist the Creator in the preservation of human life? Indeed, anything less would rob the physician of commitment and dedication and would debase the ideals of this chosen vocation.

The Destructive Power of Rejection[1]

Generations ago, the "bedside manner" was considered integral to the physician's treatment of patients. This "technique," is still a very necessary part of the healing process. This "tool," namely the use of words, proves time and again to be just what the patient needs to bring about a successful cure.

It is very likely that words of rejection are one of the prime causes for emotional illness, for crimes, for breakups and should be listed among the greatest of killers and the greatest of sins.

As rejection destroys and acceptance creates, it is imperative that words be carefully selected and prayerfully expressed so that those hearing will be comforted and filled with strength.

History has proven that through words of kindness, hope has been given to those in despair, sinners have been transformed to saints, and greatness has been instilled in those suffering from self-alienation.

No one should ever underestimate the power of affirmation and how these words expressed with heartfelt love and prayer can, through the Divine Physician, translate from sickness into health. When St. Peter saw the man crippled in the temple, he said, "I have neither silver nor gold, but what I do have I give you: in the name of Jesus Christ the Nazorean,

---

[1] Catholic Physicians' Guild (1976) "Message From the Spiritual Advisor," The Linacre Quarterly: Vol. 43: No. 4, Article 2

[rise and] walk."[2] Calling on Him, believing in Him, yes, in a "bedside manner" talking about Him, heals. Miracles do occur.

Since words heard and accepted can cause one to conceive goodness, surely the physician speaking through the inspiration of the Spirit has much more than his science to heal the sick and disturbed.

---

[2] Acts 3:6

Curing With Words[1]

While visiting a patient at the hospital, one could visualize a physician thinking, "I hope the patient is asleep when I get to the room; I hardly know what to say that will be acceptable."

The dilemma as to when, what, and how much to tell a person who is ill must be a frequent and unpleasant experience, especially when it is a serious condition. Yet, the traditional "bedside manner" which brought physicians great fame in the past, could still be very relevant and meaningful in these extremely busy days. For the patients who are wondering about their health, the evenings are long, and worry may cause frustration and affect health in unforeseen ways.

While the doctor in past decades did not have the technological knowledge and equipment of today, the physician always has the art of curing with words, as well as medicine. Jesus said, "One does not live by bread alone, but by every WORD [emphasis added] that comes forth from the mouth of God."[2] Physicians take the place of God's Son in their priestly role of curing, healing, comforting, and consoling their sisters and brothers in need.

A Catholic physician should not be embarrassed to ask suffering patients for prayers. Words uttered in pain,

---

[1] Catholic Physicians' Guild (1975) "Moderator's Page," The Linacre Quarterly: Vol. 42: No. 4, Article 2
[2] Mt 4: 4

like those of Jesus on the Cross, when uplifted in prayer have a value beyond the comprehension of humankind, for they reflect a personal union with the redemptive suffering of Christ which leads to Eternal Life.

The mystery of pain can hardly be explained. Yet the sick person may know this is a special calling. Just as there are some called to preach and others to perform apostolic works, those who are ill have a call to use their suffering, as did Christ, in the mystery of reparation for sin.

Combining the technical with comforting words makes the physician's visit to the patient not only welcomed, but meaningful. It is an opportunity to witness the presence of the gospel in a very real sense. The patient then becomes more than a client: they are brothers and sisters in Christ.

Blessed is the Catholic physician who is privileged to use words of healing and to see the profession as a vocation: an opportunity to become a messenger from God to do good for those who suffer. Surely those who suffer must be special, for God called His own Son to do the same.

Suffering and Success[1]

SUCCESS is something most people strive for. For many, it is a dream of a "better tomorrow."

For the Christian, the ultimate in success is to be welcomed into that new home, called Paradise, and enjoy the kingdom of the Lord for all eternity. However, before this happens, each person is often challenged with a "cross" of struggles and suffering.

Among the greatest obstacles in journeying through life is pain. For the Christian, pain, be it physical, emotional, psychological, or spiritual, is part of that mystery of being united with Jesus crucified.

The Sacred Congregation for the Doctrine of the Faith stated, "According to Christian teaching, suffering, especially suffering during the last moments of life, has a special place in God's saving plan; it is in fact a sharing in Christ's passion and a union with the redeeming sacrifice which He offered in obedience to the Father's will."[2]

Jesus encountered many persons with varied illnesses throughout His public life. Bartimaeus, the man born blind, the ten lepers, the woman with a hemorrhage, and Magdalen with her seven demons are but a few mentioned in the New Testament who experienced

---

[1] Lorenzetti, Dino (1982) "Message from the Spiritual Advisor," The Linacre Quarterly: Vol. 49: No. 3, Article 2
[2] Sacred Congregation for the Doctrine of the Faith: Declaration on Euthanasia, Part III, May 1980

fear, pain, and depression. As they had put their faith in Christ, they were uplifted; their handicaps became their victories.

When Dismas, the thief nailed to the cross next to Jesus on the hill of Calvary, was condemned by his community, they saw him as a "loser," rightly condemned to die. However, in the eyes of Jesus, he was indeed a "winner": he is the only person in all of Scripture who was canonized as a saint by Jesus, Himself. Our Lord said, "Today, you will be with Me in Paradise." Success in suffering.

Suffering patients need to be given hope, to be told they are loved and that their pain has meaning, that they have been called to a special apostolate which brings them into intimacy with Jesus' passion and cross, then ultimately to His resurrection.

The gospels have many examples of how Christ manifested His love to the suffering and the gospels have given us hope and the healing perspective of success.

You, as a physician, are another Christ. Like Jesus, look patiently at those whose health has failed and uplift them to success. Let them know their extraordinary worth. Let them feel very much needed and know that their pain is real prayer. Let them know that their sufferings are not in vain but that, like Dismas, they are on the cross next to Jesus, and in His sight, they are winners. They are truly victorious.

The Supernatural Power of Healing[1]

Years ago, I was challenged with a provocative question, "Why would anyone want to consult a priest if he was in crisis?" Not knowing what the precise answer would be, I asked some married couples at a seminar if they could help me with an appropriate answer. Much to my chagrin, one woman told me, "the priest is the only person I know who could verbalize a response to any problem I might have," and she saw him as God speaking directly to her. This surprising response shocked me into the realization that I'd better be mighty careful what I say and do.

I was then reminded of a true story of a priest who was visiting in Ireland. After he ignored a woman begging for alms, she sternly looked at him and said, "Well, then, Father, may I have your blessing, for you see, you have the power, but I have the faith."

The physician is regarded as the person gifted with superpowers and the patient comes with hope and expectation that, through the doctor, the crisis of illness will be changed to the restoration of health.

The physician often feels inadequate, especially if the illness is beyond the wisdom of science. The limit of one's expertise, the restricted knowledge of certain diseases, the mystery of the process of healing, all

---

[1] Lorenzetti, Dino J. (1983) "Message from the Spiritual Advisor: The Physician's Skills," The Linacre Quarterly: Vol. 50: No. 4, Article 2

seem to restrain the physician's ability to practice medical art with confidence.

However, the grace of the Lord "flows" through you and as instruments of God's peace, you are invited to the impossible. In God, all things are possible, and there is great rejoicing in seeing the glory of God manifested in our weak nature.

You are called to believe – to witness love in action, to be a people of hope for a new tomorrow. God gives you His strength as you put your faith in Him. As a physician, you are given extraordinary opportunities to perform miracles of healing through His power of grace.

Your speech, your touch, your advice, your knowledge, your skills – but above all your faith – make it possible. You are Christ's hands among the sick and needy. Therefore, your profession should never be taken for granted, nor be damaged by pride, arrogance, nor money. Yours is a supernatural gift: a blessed sacrament, a profession which has power like a missile containing nuclear energy which can be used to soar to the outer planets or used for destruction and annihilation.

As we are all called to be, you are another Christ: walking, talking, and healing those who believe. To be effective, you, like Christ, must pray to the Father with faith. Your vocation is awesome ... scary ... beautiful. You are indeed among God's chosen.

Our Disease: Lack of Self-Worth[1]

George Gallup, Jr, in his report on "Religion in America," stated that the levels of self-esteem are low for many persons.[2] The biggest disease in America today is not cancer or heart disease, but a person's lack of self-worth.

There are many persons who are lonely, unemployed, feel unwanted, depressed, and homeless. There are also great numbers who see themselves as failures in their marriage, in their work, and in their studies. To ease their pain, some have resorted to drugs, alcohol, overeating, divorce, violence, and even suicide. These effects are interpreted as the results of human weakness, or by some, as the evil of our fallen nature, namely original sin. However it is viewed, it is important that every individual be open to examine his or her own negativity.

The physician's presence in this "holy" place is most valuable and its worth indisputable when examining the patient asking for help. Armed with medical knowledge, words of encouragement, counsel, affirmation, and inspiration, the physician's treatment becomes more than therapeutic; it becomes a "healing ointment."

---

[1] Lorenzetti, Dino J. (1986) "Message from the Spiritual Advisor: Lack of Self-Worth," The Linacre Quarterly: Vol. 53: No. 1, Article 2
[2] Gallup G. Religion in America. The ANNALS of the American Academy of Political and Social Science. 1985

The physician of faith believes that where two or more are gathered in God's name, Jesus is present. So, be prepared to uplift one who is "down and out" and be open to God's grace working through you.

In the life of Our Blessed Mother, this experience of extraordinary grace took place through her. When she was called to become the Mother of God, she immediately responded to serve as His maid. Her answer to the angel's invitation: "Behold, I am the handmaid of the Lord. May it be done to me according to your word."[3] Through Mary's faith and humility, salvation history became a reality.

It is through the physician that God's grace becomes efficacious when, as a servant, the doctor is open to our sisters and brothers in pain. The physician becomes empowered, through His Spirit, to raise the debilitated to strength, restore the sick to health, and direct the astray to sainthood.

In this paradox, your humility as a servant, exalts you as a doctor of grandeur. Your mission to serve becomes your honor to "treat" Christ, as His words are: "Amen, I say to you, whatever you did for one of these least brothers of mine, you did for me."[4] In giving your time to the troubled and those with lack of self-worth, you are raised with them to new life.

---

[3] Lk 1: 38
[4] Mt 25: 40

Section 5: What is Truth in a Secular Society?

Courage in a Secular Society[1]

No generation has ever challenged the physician of faith as the people of this modern age. With statutory controls over medical practice, with extraordinary insurance premiums for malpractice, with difficult ethical questions to resolve in biogenetics, with tremendous family stresses in the home, the doctor is compelled to act in a seemingly uncompromising position.

The inability to freely exercise this sacred vocation without reprisal is indisputable. Yet in spite of the ever-new obstacles in the path towards caring for the sick, you must proceed with confidence, recognizing that the Holy Spirit, the Spirit of healing, is within you.

The prophet Isaiah proclaims, "Strengthen hands that are feeble, make firm knees that are weak, Say to the fearful of heart: Be strong, do not fear!"[2]

To have courage and speak out, at the risk of being ridiculed by one's colleagues, to the doctrines that proclaim sanctity of life, shows that you have faith. To suffer what is seemingly humiliation when in disagreement with famed popular scientists on doctrines of truth, places you among the blessed. To see

---

[1] Lorenzetti, Dino J. (1986) "Message from the Spiritual Advisor: Modern Age Challenges Physicians," The Linacre Quarterly: Vol. 53: No. 2, Article 2
[2] Is 35:3-4

the solution to the problem, not necessarily as the secularist in the light of humanitarianism, but as a person of faith who sees the solution in conformity with the laws of the Creator, is to share the vision of the prophet.

In defending one's position courageously, it is important at all times: that the individual be a person of prayer; that the words used when praying and speaking to God are in keeping with actions towards our sisters and brothers in need of medical services; that charity, compassion, and patience be especially among the virtues that exemplify the physician as a believer; that the medical practice has the courage to witness faith by the way patients are treated; that, as a physician of faith, there is but one goal in mind: the salvation of the immortal soul.

There will always be a distinction between the physician and the physician of faith. The latter has more to offer than scientific medical knowledge and care. The faithful person sees each individual as a sister and brother in Christ, every human being made to the image and likeness of God, every person as destined for eternal life. The physician looks inward and sees one called to heal, privileged to touch that debilitated patient.

May God the Father reward you for your dedication towards His people and may He praise you as He did His Son, Jesus: namely, in claiming you as beloved, and one in whom He is well pleased.

Truth and the Physician[1]

One of the most difficult challenges in life is facing the truth. This is indeed painful at times, yet this is how we profess our integrity as sacred persons.

There is no compromise with truth! IT IS! For example, human life is in the fertilized ovum; many would like to think otherwise, but that is the fact.

For a physician to defend the truth is to undertake one of the most troublesome realities in this profession. Many medical colleagues are "chained" to programs that promote an untruth: they search endlessly for "truth," or rather, for answers that best suit their mode of behavior.

When conscious of a procedure that is contrary to the Hippocratic Oath, or dispensing medication for social reasons that do harm to the body, or when advocating legislation not beneficial to the total well-being of an individual, there is dishonesty. The truth is suppressed, goodness ignored, and the concern becomes selfish rather than loving – the patient becomes a victim wounded by the healer when traveling in life to the final goal.

You are well aware of what happens when dealing with patients who resist and wrestle with the truth. They develop all kinds of anxieties, frustrations and "hang-ups." Nature seems to torture them for they know they

---

[1] Lorenzetti, Dino J. (1979) "Message From the Spiritual Advisor," The Linacre Quarterly: Vol. 46: No. 4, Article 2

have deceived themselves. Speaking untruths is an abuse of the precious gift of speech – a gift given only to humans – and this gift is perverted.

Pilate, when seeing Truth, asked the question of Jesus, "What is truth?"[2] Pilate was perplexed, and rightly so. He had a face-to-face conflict between his vocation and his voice which led, as you know, to the "destruction" of Truth.

As Catholic physicians, there is no need to be afraid of speaking loudly and clearly for God is with you. In the sacred scriptures, there are more than three hundred passages written on the importance of truth. In the Gospel of John, Jesus proclaims: "you will know the truth, and the truth will set you free."[3]

Jesus teaches, "I am the way, the TRUTH [emphasis added] and the life."[4] Yes, it is through Him on our pilgrim journey that we stay on the right road which leads to new life. For the traveler who does not know the "way" and is given wrong information, it becomes mighty hard, if not impossible, to arrive at the proper destination. As men and women of God, instruments and prophets of His truth, you are the voice that can show the way, thus directing His people to life and holiness. "Through all generations your truth endures."[5]

---

[2] Jn 18: 38
[3] Jn 8: 32
[4] Jn 14: 6
[5] Ps 119: 90

Apostolic Mission on the Right to Life[1]

Catholic physicians are continually challenged by their own colleagues as they practice their apostolic mission of teaching and healing.

Knowledge of the glaring data proving serious consequences associated with the use of oral contraceptives and intrauterine devices compels the physician to speak up and discourage their use. As objections are voiced to contraceptives, abortion, sterilization, and euthanasia, the physician becomes an unpopular advocate, especially if the remarks are directed against governmental legislation or social programs.

Unfortunately, some have compromised the principles of their noble profession for other values. They have surrendered their "birth right" and abrogated responsibilities of their profession to others. The blaring noise of health authorities and the pressure of interest groups sometimes "out shout" the voice of the Shepherd who cries, "Follow Me."

In London, the Right Reverend Patrick Casey, Bishop of Brentwood, cautioned the European Federation of Catholic Physicians at their Third Congress[2] that

---

[1] Catholic Physicians' Guild (1976) "Moderator's Page," The Linacre Quarterly: Vol. 43: No. 3, Article 2
[2] London, England; European federation 'FEAMC' Third World Congress, 1976

"physicians should work hand in hand with legislators, but NOT hand in glove with them."

May those physicians who are temporarily discouraged recall the words of St. Paul: "...stand firm in one spirit, with one mind struggling together for the faith of the gospel, not intimidated in any way by your opponents. This is proof to them of destruction, but of your salvation. And this is God's doing."[3]

Listen and obey the voice of the Church. Be strengthened for the promise of Christ: "I will be with you always."[4]

---

[3] Phil 1: 27-28
[4] Mt 28: 20

The Value of Life[1]

What value, life!

When Jesus brought His dear friend Lazarus back to life, He signed his own death warrant, for His disciple, John, tells us that it was "from that day on they planned to kill him."[2] The price Jesus paid for Lazarus' life was His own. With tears in His eyes, Jesus went to the tomb to bring Lazarus to life. Physicians often see an expectant mother in tears as she anticipates life from her womb. Yet moments of distress are not lasting, for soon her weeping bursts into joy as she sees what God has brought.

The mystery of God's creation which marvelously knit the infant in her womb can never be realized or decided upon with science alone, for the value of a life is not a statistic. Life is a sacred gift given by God: a gift that becomes a witness, a brother or sister, a friend, a prophet unique to all others with a hope and a vision to greatness. Perhaps the individual becomes an inventor, a scientist, or theologian with the wisdom to resolve the ills plaguing society and restores a people to happiness.

The book of Genesis declares that what God created is GOOD. As the genetic engineers announce their great progress and fears, scientists are urged to be cautious

---

[1] Lorenzetti, Dino J. (1977) "Message From the Spiritual Advisor," The Linacre Quarterly: Vol. 44: No. 4, Article 2
[2] Jn 11: 53

in their experimentations as they fringe on the very creation of life that is GOOD. The healing physician allies with the power of divine goodness. In caring, loving, and curing the life created by God, the physician becomes mysteriously united with Him.

Therefore, life is never to be "tampered with," demeaned, destroyed or disposed of – only enriched. Each conception is a new life that never existed before. From the moment there is a child in a womb, there is a loving person with fears, expectations, and joys. This conception becomes a new "concept" and the woman is chosen by God to bear life, to bring forth a child with a potential to continue its existence from generation to generation.

The physician values this precious vocation of working with God, the Creator of His people, and giving them the benefits of medical talents. In fact, the doctor may be put "on the line" by accepting risks, criticism, and often loss of financial security, as the life of another is lifted up. In essence, like Jesus, the physician speaks up – not in bringing life from the *tomb*, but life from the *womb*. In so doing, it does not matter what happens, for in love the doctor's life is buried so another may live.

A physician is special: the mission of Jesus is continued in bringing forth life.

The Absolute Evil of Abortion[1]

When Peter and the Apostles were challenged before the Sanhedrin and the high priest, they were told: "We gave you strict orders [did we not?] to stop teaching in that name." Peter, however, responded, "We must obey God rather than men."[2]

Today that same message is relevant to all persons of faith who believe in the Word of God. The fifth commandment of the Decalogue consists of only four words: "Thou shalt not kill" – words that are clear, distinct, precise, and in no way disputable. Yet society has ignored the divine mandate and has legislated laws in the name of some social or economic "good" which are in direct violation of what God has commanded.

With federal and state legislation, abortions became legalized. Euthanasia was the next target with the intent to lure the sympathy and approval of the general public into this style of mercy killing.

The killing of the body or the spirit of any person brings with it curses and condemnations. Jesus warns us: "Things that cause sin will inevitably occur, but woe to the person through whom they occur. It would be better for him if a millstone were put around his

---

[1] Lorenzetti, Dino J. (1986) "Message from the Spiritual Advisor: Killing Brings Condemnation," The Linacre Quarterly: Vol. 53: No. 4, Article 2
[2] Acts 5: 28-29 *and* (1987) "Physicians and Their Faith," Vol. 54: No. 3, Article 2

neck and he be thrown into the sea than for him to cause one of these little ones to sin. Be on your guard."[3]

For the physician believing in the God who gave Moses the Ten Commandments, and for the Christian who upholds in faith the teachings of Jesus, certainly the direct and deliberate killing of an innocent person will be subjected to the judgment of God.

Cain's question, "Am I my brother's keeper?"[4] is still the same for all those who claim society's laws are superior to the Divine law of life.

After being questioned and flogged by the Sanhedrin, the Apostles left "rejoicing that they had been found worthy to suffer dishonor for the sake of the name."[5]

Since the legalization of abortion, Catholic physicians have been called upon to pay a great price for their faith. For many, promotions were denied and their income drastically reduced, and for others, their witness to the faith is ridiculed as they voice their strong objections to the killing of the innocent child in the mother's womb.

Dear God ... May the ill-treatment received in defending your laws and praise of Your name not bring us discouragement but joy, peace, and new life, as was given to the Apostles. Amen.

---

[3] Lk 17: 1-2
[4] Gen 4: 9
[5] Acts 5: 41

Hero or Scapegoat?[1]

We live in a society that daily creates heroes and scapegoats. We wait for the latest newscast to see who are the winners and losers of the day: political success or failure, the outcome of the races, the advances or declines on the market, or the final scores of the games played. As human beings interested in the adventures and challenges of our fellow citizens, we vicariously sit back and observe as "armchair critics," expressing our praise or disapproval of what we see or hear.

Unfortunately, the physician can be looked upon in pretty much the same way. Either the doctor is a hero: a great person, a savior, a genius; or, a scapegoat: the fall guy, a loser, incompetent. If the doctor speaks up for the truth, sometimes the label is "fool." It is paradoxical that many times the doctor is judged as both: hero and scapegoat, just as Jesus was during the week of His crucifixion. The crowds hailed Him as a king on Palm Sunday and as a criminal on Good Friday: "like a lamb led to slaughter."[2]

Heroes have strength which is overpowering and their faults go unnoticed, whereas scapegoats are vulnerable since they carry fault and blame. Often, they are accused with just enough truth to make the

---

[1] Lorenzetti, Dino J. (1980) "Message From the Spiritual Advisor," The Linacre Quarterly: Vol. 47: No. 3, Article 2
[2] Is 53: 7

accusation sound credible and thus they become victims for attack.

Jesus is the "Lamb of God" (the scapegoat) who takes away the sins of the world. Yes, He is our hero; He has mercy on us. Yet the price of His life, carrying the fault and blame upon himself, is what brought us salvation. Physicians, like the Divine Healer, deal with sickness which is frequently equated as the visible sign of disorder in the person. Healing is the taking away of the disorder, the sickness, and is the restoration to health.

Today many Catholic physicians can identify with Jesus as the price of giving over their lives is what brings healing. The doctor has mercy on the sick and can relate to his brother and sister in pain. As a person of faith, blessings are received as faith is visible in the work.

The prophet Jeremiah extols, "Cursed is the man who trusts in human beings... Blessed are those who trust in the Lord."[3] How do you see yourself? If one in Christ, you could be a scapegoat/fool to the world, but more important, you are the hero/saint in His Kingdom.

---

[3] Jer 17: 5,7

Pragmatism May Facilitate Evil[1]

Before our first parents committed original sin, the tempter, the prince of devils, had already fallen from the grace of God and scored his victory on the goodness of God's love. This is described in the Book of Genesis, the story of creation, when God created the world and the first couple. It was from these earliest days that evil has tormented humankind.

A pragmatic perspective can be dangerous and lead us into darkness. Pragmatism can teach us to discard, reject, or destroy all that is no longer useful. Tragically, this philosophy of life has gone far beyond such things as furniture and appliances. It has invaded the very realm of the divine, destroying the God's gifts which He designed in love for us.

Through scientific experimentation, love is absent from the act of procreation as children are "made" in a dish. With the killing of unwanted babies in their mother's womb, God's goodness is frustrated, and evil is perpetuated!

In Jesus' parables, there is a gap of time from the moment of planting the seed to its harvest. That time is for the minerals in the soil and the sunshine and rain to do their work so that the seed will grow and bear fruit. St. Paul describes it this way: "I planted,

---

[1] Lorenzetti, Dino J. (1987) "Message from the Spiritual Advisor: From the Beginning: Evil," The Linacre Quarterly: Vol. 54: No. 2, Article 2

Apollos watered, but God caused the growth."[2] Harvesting requires time, God's timing.

But the pragmatist may push forward his own way rather than calling on God's guidance. God's grace is more than important: it is essential.

In witnessing His Gospel, a Eucharistic physician is infused with the blood of Christ. So as Jesus overcame the prince of d(evil)s, so, too, the person of faith may do the same.

The Blessed Virgin, Queen of Angels, has supremacy over all spirits, even those who have fallen from on high and "roam the world seeking the ruin of souls." Confident of her protection, no one need be afraid, but rather uplifted with the prayer that "it has never been known that anyone who invoked your help was left unaided."[3] We also pray the Lord will deliver us from evil, every time we recite The Lord's Prayer. There is much protection for us, if we seek it.

Pity the pragmatists when life seems "useless," while the faithful are blessed with an eternal perspective and rejoice in His promise of new life.

---

[2] 1 Cor 3: 6

[3] The Memorare: "Remember, O most gracious Virgin Mary, that never was it known that anyone who fled to thy protection, implored thy help, or sought thy intercession was left unaided. Inspired with this confidence, I fly to thee, O Virgin of virgins, my Mother; to thee do I come; before thee I stand, sinful and sorrowful. O Mother of the Word Incarnate, despise not my petitions, but in thy mercy hear and answer me. Amen."

Obstacles in Legal Regulations[1]

With governmental intervention in medicine, there appears to be a syndrome in our society which makes it awkward for dedicated physicians to extend courtesies and charity to clients who call on them. In years past, it was easier for a physician to render services to those in discomfort without the mandated record-keeping and bureaucratic overseeing in the healing process. It is certainly with justifiable concern that physicians, now more than ever, observe medical, hospital, and legal regulations in compliance with their code of ethics, so as to avoid being penalized for their actions. The simplicity of curing with love and restoring the sick to good health seems hampered because of the "structure."

The Catholic physician could interpret this troublesome "red tape" into a positive mode of action, if this time-consuming and painstaking process was deliberated as a way to assist the patient seeking help. There is a strong sense of dignity in most individuals being serviced through varied public medical insurance programs. Patients are willing to give what little they have and hope that, in participating with the doctor, there will arise the miracle of returning to good health. It reminds me of our offering of the gifts of bread and wine (small as that may be) with the expectation, through the miracle of grace, they will

---

[1] Lorenzetti, Dino J. (1977) "Message from the Spiritual Advisor," The Linacre Quarterly: Vol. 44: No. 1, Article 2

become the Body and Blood of Jesus, remitting our sins.

As a person of faith, each physician is anxious to give this gift of "new" life to the person afflicted with sickness and disease. The physician shares in a sublime way the divine life as the weak and oppressed, who come pleading for healing powers, are restored. The sick person exposes vulnerability with whatever offering or stipend can be offered and asks in return to be restored to health.

The Catholic physician continues the mission of Jesus in this ministry of healing. The poor are often reluctant to approach one who could be their help. Be very sensitive not to scare away the sick desiring your services. Posters, cards, or notices (no matter how polite they may read) stating that certain types of insurance benefits are not accepted could create a deeper problem, one of rejection. Share willingly your talents with those seeking comfort and strength. Then, on that last day, you will find no exclusion notice barring you from a warm welcome from the Divine Savior. "Amen, I say to you, whatever you did for one of these least brothers of mine, you did for me."[2] Yes, Jesus is asking you to be His doctor – to care for Him.

---

[2] Mt 25: 40

Working Toward a Dream: Medicine and the Law[1]

Every physician's ideal is to accomplish good, restore the sick to health, and bring joy and comfort to the hearts of patients. Perhaps there is a hope that, through your tireless studies and with the grace of God, a technique or procedure might be developed which would help fellow colleagues in the science of healing.

The doctors' heroes are those extraordinary persons such as Dr. Louis Pasteur, Dr. Jonas Salk, Dr. Elizabeth Blackwell (first woman in US to earn a medical degree) and others whose contributions to the world community are truly legacies of greatness.

Today, many physicians are stifled with fear as they recognize that actions intended as good may lead to a malpractice suit. The end result from such a legal contest can be totally damaging to the practitioner whose whole life is dedicated to helping others.

It can be difficult for legislatures to enact law which anticipates the effect on individuals and the result may be losing sight of human values. In their struggle to rationalize truth into neat pragmatic legal formulas that will be socially acceptable, legislatures witness the individual victimized in the process. The judicial branch has similar issues.

---

[1] Lorenzetti, Dino J. (1980) "Message From the Spiritual Advisor," The Linacre Quarterly: Vol. 47: No. 4, Article 2

A clear example is the Supreme Court consistently denying the rights of the child within the womb, yet no physician can deny that life from conception is human. After all these years, the struggle for the protection of life continues to be a relevant and pressing issue.

Such controversies can lead to a schism between physicians and lawyers. The result is devastating to all of society. Both professions may find themselves totally at odds. Courts, while deciding lucrative claims, make fine distinctions on such sensitive issues as the rights of the human body vs. human rights. Courts and legislatures consider such issues: "Which is evil, killing the person or keeping him alive?"; "Why is the brain wave of the fetus not recognized as a human person whereas the brain wave of the human out of the womb is?"; "When does death occur?" Problems become even more complex with the intervention of third parties. Thus, professional counselors are faced with these issues as well as business groups such as insurance companies who decide "how much" and "to whom" payments are to be made for the "human services."

How can we better dialogue on these issues? Can we have a chance to reflect, to call on the Spirit, and invite the community to contribute its input? Can we accept the challenge by dialoguing with lawyers and physicians, as well as theologians and counselors?

The medical profession is truly a noble one and its members are genuinely needed and respected. However, the fear of "being sued" for doing one's job to the best of one's ability should not preoccupy the mind so that it becomes the most perplexing problem of this vocation.

As a people of faith, believing in the work of the Spirit, you need not fear. Continue your mission of healing while striving with other professions for better cooperation and understanding. Exercise your skills fearlessly for the good of humankind and encourage counselors, as well as theologians, to be peacemakers who assist the physician/patient relationship toward harmony.

These can indeed be troublesome times and, with all dedicated people involved in human services, the wholistic individual is of paramount importance. Working together toward this same objective, all of society can be beneficiaries of the arts and sciences, of law and theology, and of the best that God has given to us in His universe.

Is this a dream? Perhaps so. But, before there is change, you must first have a dream.

About the Author

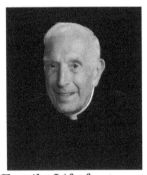

For almost 70 years, Rev. Msgr. Dino J. Lorenzetti has been a well-known and much-loved priest of the Diocese of Buffalo. Born and raised in Buffalo, NY, he was ordained to the priesthood in 1953 after serving our country for three years during WWII. He was Director of the Diocesan Office of Family Life for twenty years and served as a pastor for twenty-seven years. Additionally, he was heavily involved in the Foundation for International Cooperation (FIC), the Diocesan Guild of Catholic Physicians, Interfaith Committee, Rachel Project, and spiritual advisor for the National Federation of Catholic Physicians Guilds (now, Catholic Medical Association). Pope St. Paul VI appointed him as Ecclesiastical Assistant to the International Federation of Catholic Medical Associations and he served in this role under Pope St. John Paul II, as well. In this capacity, he was blessed to be honored with Saint Mother Teresa in Mumbai, India. In 2010, was the recipient of Most Rev. Edward U. Kmiec Bishop's Medal. Since then, he has authored three other books: *Agony of Betrayal, Addio: See You in Heaven,* and *Seven Minute Homilies.* Msgr. Lorenzetti turns 100 years old in July 2021 and continues his "retirement" by enjoying life and remaining active in ministry in the Diocese of Buffalo.